THE

Natural Health

GUIDE TO

Antioxidants

■

Supplements to
Fight Disease and
Maintain Optimal Health

NANCY BRUNING
and the Editors of *Natural Health*

BANTAM BOOKS
NEW YORK · TORONTO · LONDON · SYDNEY · AUCKLAND

THE NATURAL HEALTH GUIDE TO ANTIOXIDANTS

A Bantam Book / April 1994

Though this book presents the research suggesting the efficacy of antioxidants in preventing disease, it is not intended to provide medical advice or to substitute for the advice of your personal physician or primary care practitioner. The reader should regularly consult a physician in matters relating to his or her health and individual needs, particularly in respect to any symptoms which may require diagnosis or medical attention. Naturally, if you are on a prescription drug, you must not stop taking it without first consulting with your doctor. If you are concerned your physician might not be aware of or fully educated about the possible benefits of antioxidants, bring this book along with you to the doctor's office.

ISBN 0-553-56579-6

Published simultaneously in the United States and Canada

Bantam Books are published by Bantam Books, a division of Bantam Doubleday Dell Publishing Group, Inc. Its trademark, consisting of the words "Bantam Books" and the portrayal of a rooster, is Registered in U.S. Patent and Trademark Office and in other countries. Marca Registrada. Bantam Books, 1540 Broadway, New York, New York 10036.

PRINTED IN THE UNITED STATES OF AMERICA

OPM   0 9 8 7 6 5 4 3 2 1

THE EVIDENCE IS IN . . .

- University of Texas researchers report that antioxidant nutrients inhibit plaque formation in the bloodstream, a factor in heart disease.
- At the Salk Institute for Biological Studies researchers discover evidence suggesting that vitamin E combats the death of brain cells, delaying age-related brain damage.
- Harvard Medical School studies find that people who take beta carotene and vitamin E supplements have fewer heart attacks and strokes.
- University of Washington researchers develop a test to identify women who may be able to prevent breast cancer through antioxidant therapy.

The Natural Health Guide to Antioxidants covers the latest exciting discoveries into antioxidants and how these vitamins and minerals can prevent or minimize the damage that may lead to accelerated aging and dozens of degenerative diseases such as cancer, heart disease, arthritis, immune disease, and cataracts.

It provides you with guidelines, based on what prominent researchers and clinicians are saying, about how to create your own antioxidant defense program through eating right and exercising. It also recommends the safe dose range for supplements, based on research data and observations. And it takes a peek into the future to a time when antioxidant therapy may be routinely used to prevent and treat diseases at their earliest stages.

**THIS IS A BOOK
YOU CAN'T AFFORD TO MISS!**

Acknowledgments

■

The author would like to thank the following for contributing their time and sharing their expertise during the preparation of this book:

ANTHONY L. ALMADA, M.Sc., Director of Research and Development, Rainbow Light Nutritional Systems

ADRIANNE BENDICH, Ph.D., Clinical Research Scientist, Human Nutrition Research, Hoffmann-La Roche, Inc.

JEFFREY S. BLAND, Ph.D., educator, founder and CEO of HealthComm, and Senior Investigator, American Association of Clinical Scientists

JEFFREY BLUMBERG, Ph.D., Associate Director and Professor, Human Nutrition Research Center on Aging, Tufts University

MARY BURNETT, Director of Public Affairs, Council for Responsible Nutrition

STEPHEN LEVINE, Ph.D., President, Nutricology/Allergy Research Group

SHARI LIEBERMAN, Ph.D., clinical nutritionist

DONALD MALINS, Ph.D., director of Molecular Epidemiology, the Pacific Northwest Research Foundation, Seattle, WA

ROBERT McCALEB, herb educator and President, Herb Research Foundation

WILLIAM PRYOR, Ph.D., Director, Biodynamics Institute, Louisiana State University

HARI SHARMA, M.D., Professor of Pathology and Director, Cancer Prevention and Natural Products Research, the Ohio State University

Thanks are also due to Marilyn McGregor, Christine Moen, and Stephen Wheeler for their research and editorial assistance.

Contents

∎

Introduction

■

For the first time, a study has shown that taking vitamin and mineral supplements can reduce the cancer death rate in a large population sample.

In the study, published in *The Journal of the National Cancer Institute* in September, 1993, a team of researchers from China and from the U.S.'s National Cancer Institute divided approximately 30,000 people living in Linxian County in Henan Province of north-central China into eight groups. Cancer death rates in Linxian are among the highest in the world. For five years, seven of the groups were given different regimens of vitamins and minerals in amounts one to two times the doses recommended in the U.S. The eighth group received dummy pills.

Overall death rates of those who took the vitamins and minerals were less than the rates of those who took the dummy pills. One particular regimen consisting of beta-carotene (a precursor of vitamin A), vitamin E, and the mineral selenium reduced the death rate by 13 percent. These three nutrients are among those known to act as antioxidants and curb the activity of disease-causing free radicals. The amounts of vitamin E and selenium given were equal to the U.S. Recommended Allowances, and the amount of beta-carotene given was roughly twice the amount generally recommended in the U.S.

Researchers said that the results give hope that nutritional supplements can reduce cancer death rates, but they urged caution in extrapolating the results to the American population. As a group, the people of Linxian are undernourished, which is not the case in the U.S., and that may account for their extremely high death rates (in the case of esophageal cancer, about 50 times the U.S. death rate). The people of Linxian also consume certain foods, like pickled vegetables, that are believed to increase the risk of some cancers.

Officials at the National Cancer Institute said that studies of the effects of vitamins on U.S. population groups are presently underway, but results won't be known for at least several years.

In what a prominent researcher has called "the second wave of vitamin research," scientists are supplying solid evidence that vitamins are more powerful than we ever imagined. New research supports the view that while eating in accordance with the Recommended Dietary Allowances (RDAs) may prevent obvious deficiency diseases, like scurvy, these standards are obsolete and have little to do with today's concerns about optimum health.

Many scientists believe they may have a found a common underlying biochemical mechanism that links many seemingly unrelated health conditions. Research in biochemistry, epidemiology, nutrition, immunology, neurology, gerontology, pathology, oncology, and ophthalmology is providing clues as to why we age and get sick—and how we can slow or head off these processes. Findings in these many disparate fields are laying the foundation for a whole new way of thinking about disease prevention. They are also providing us with the tools to help us prevent and in some cases stop the progression of heart disease and cancer—the two major killers in our culture. And they are helping us understand how to maintain optimum health well into old age.

The research centers on a group of compounds that are known as antioxidants. These compounds—common vitamins like C and E, beta-carotene (the chemical parent of vitamin A), minerals like selenium and zinc, and other substances like green tea and Pycnogenol, which is derived from the bark of pine trees—may one day be routinely used to prevent a wide array of diseases and conditions ranging from cataracts and wrinkles to cancer and heart disease. According to one researcher, studies to date have identified more than 60 health conditions that may be prevented or treated with antioxidant supplementation, and "new diseases are regularly being added to the list."

Our bodies use antioxidants to stay healthy by deploying them against *free radicals,* highly reactive atoms or molecules that have lost one electron and are aggressively seeking a replacement. Free radicals are a by-product of normal metabolism in cells, such as the burning of food for energy, or the fighting of infection. They are formed in our bodies when, for example, molecules of fat react with oxygen in a process similar to that which turns fat rancid, or makes metal rust. These harmful molecules are also formed by exposure to toxic environmental pollutants in our food and water, and in our air from car exhaust, tobacco smoke, and ozone; exposure to radiation, insecticides, and excessive sunlight also leads to the formation of free radicals. Free radicals can damage our body's healthy cells in many ways, including inducing gene mutation, which sets the foundation for cancer.

We form free radicals all the time. But just as our body defends itself from viruses and bacterial infection, so it uses defense mechanisms that keep oxidation processes—or free radical formation—under control. One mechanism works by repairing the cell damage. Another intercepts, or "scavenges," free radicals before they cause harm. This "quenching" of free radicals is the role of antioxidants.

When we succumb to disease, it means these normal cellular processes and safeguards are either not in place or are no longer enough to maintain health. Unfortunately, today the typical American diet contains increased amounts of fats and fewer fresh fruits and vegetables, and we are exposed to more environmental pollution than in the past; this makes our need for antioxidants to control free radicals greater than ever in the history of humankind. Yet the antioxidant content of our diets has plummeted.

This book describes the vitamins, minerals, and enzymes that work as antioxidants and help the body protect itself. Many of these substances are available in food—notably yellow, orange, and green leafy vegetables and yellow-orange fruits—but in relatively small and possibly inadequate amounts. Although many of the researchers involved in studies refrain from recommending that the general public take antioxidant supplements, most find the evidence compelling enough to take supplements themselves. A number of recent studies strongly support the role of antioxidants and disease prevention. For example:

• University of Texas researchers report that antioxidant nutrients suppress oxidation of fat particles in the bloodstream and inhibit plaque formation, a factor in heart disease.
• At the Salk Institute for Biological Studies in California, researchers have found that vitamin E may combat the death of brain cells by scavenging free radicals, thereby delaying age-related brain damage.
• Two large studies conducted at the Harvard Medical

School have found that men and women who consume high levels of beta-carotene and vitamin E have fewer heart attacks and strokes.

• Researchers at the University of Washington and the Pacific Northwest Research Foundation have developed a test that could be used to identify women at high risk of breast cancer and who may prevent the disease through antioxidant therapy.

This book covers what we know and do not know about antioxidants, and provides you with important information and guidance about how incorporating antioxidants into a sensible life-style can help protect your health. It explains what free radicals are and how antioxidants protect us from free radical damage. It discusses the evidence that certain vitamins, minerals, and other substances can, through their antioxidant capabilities, prevent or minimize the accumulated damage that may lead to accelerated aging and dozens of degenerative diseases such as cancer, heart disease, arthritis, immune disease, and cataracts.

This book also provides information on the best food sources for antioxidants as well as the safe dose range for supplements, based on research data and observations. It explains why you need to pay attention to other factors that contribute to free radical formation in the body, such as fatty food, alcohol, air pollution, and exposure to radiation, tobacco smoke, and sunlight. It gives guidelines, based on what prominent researchers and clinicians are saying, about how to create your own antioxidant defense program. And finally, it takes a peek into the future—the direction that free radical research is taking and how this could improve our ability to use antioxidant therapy safely and inexpensively to prevent and treat diseases at their earliest stages.

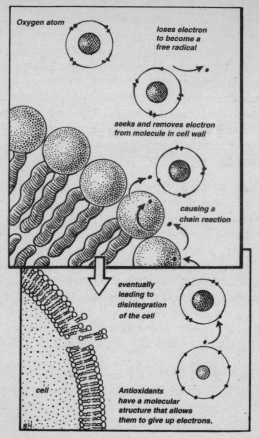

Oxygen atom

loses electron to become a free radical

seeks and removes electron from molecule in cell wall

causing a chain reaction

eventually leading to disintegration of the cell

cell

Antioxidants have a molecular structure that allows them to give up electrons.

A free radical is a molecule or atom that has lost an electron. Radicals are highly unstable and reactive, and they will seek to regain their balanced state by "stealing" an electron from a nearby molecule or atom. In stabilizing itself, the molecule creates a new unstable free radical, setting off a chain reaction. Such reactions in our cell walls may lead to a variety of chronic health problems, including cancer and heart disease.

Our bodies have the ability to "quench" free radicals with so-called antioxidants. Antioxidants are compounds that combine readily with free radicals, but do not generate additional radicals during the reaction. Our bodies manufacture antioxidants, and we can derive them from foods (notably fruits and vegetables) and supplements like vitamins A, C, and E. *(Drawing by Barbara Harmon)*

ONE

Free Radicals and Antioxidants:

A PRECARIOUS BALANCE

■

Free radicals are renegade substances that form naturally in our bodies as a by product of metabolism. As such, they are an intrinsic part of the day-to-day processes our bodies perform to survive: if we couldn't create waste products and toxins through our healthy bodily functions, we would die. Yet, if allowed to increase out of control and if not eliminated from our bodies, free radicals also have the potential to cause great harm to our cells, tissues, and organs. Fortunately, our bodies have developed a special defense system which, under normal circumstances, is designed to keep things in balance.

What's a Free Radical?

The word *radical* was first used in chemistry by Antoine Lavoisier, the founder of modern chemistry. By *radical* he meant an element that combined with oxygen in an acid. Today the term has come to mean any molecule that is missing an electron. An electron is a subatomic particle that spins in orbit around the nucleus of an atom. Electrons have either an "up" or a "down" spin, and usually come in pairs, with each partner carrying a different spin. A radical, however, is in an unbalanced, unstable state and seeks to restore its balance by completing its pair. It is said to be *reactive,* because it reacts with a nearby molecule either by "stealing" an electron or by giving away its spare.

The problem is that the action doesn't always stop there: in restoring its balance, the radical creates a new unbalanced molecule that now has to restore *its* balance by giving or taking an electron from another molecule, creating still another imbalance and setting in motion a volatile chain reaction. When the electron chain reaction involves molecules in a normal cell, the molecules may be destroyed and unable to function.

William Pryor, Ph.D., director of the Biodynamics Institute at Louisiana State University, uses the analogy of the bachelor at a dance party to explain free radical reactions. "The bachelor walks in and everybody else is coupled. In order to pair up with a woman, he has to cut in on a couple, setting loose another bachelor. That bachelor needs to cut in on another couple, and so on. To stop this process, you would have to admit an extra female. Otherwise it would go on forever.[1]

Free radicals are a good news/bad news phenomenon inside and outside the body. We've learned how to harness them to synthesize plastics. Without the action of free radicals, bread couldn't turn into crispy browned toast. We buy products containing free radicals at the drugstore, such as antifungal medicine and hydrogen peroxide, and use them to treat athlete's foot and kill bacteria. But radicals also cause great paintings to deteriorate, butter to turn rancid, rubber to turn brittle, and cars to rust.

Inside the body, runaway free radical chain reactions can sabotage our cells—the building blocks of all our tissues and organs. These reactions damage cell membranes (the thin wall that surrounds each cell), DNA (the genetic code), and proteins needed to perform essential metabolic functions. This damage in turn may lead to a host of chronic and acute health problems. Like paint, butter, and metal, our tissues deteriorate, turn "rancid," and "rust."

The Good News

Free radicals, however, are necessary for life. To understand why, we need to go back 3.5 billion years—to the genesis of life on this planet. As we now know, ultraviolet radiation from the sun forms free radicals. It is believed that free radicals produced the molecules needed in the primordial soup for the first protocells to survive. In addition, the interaction of free radicals with early cell life produced the genetic mutations required for cells to evolve into more complex and hardy life forms.

Today, most life forms on earth still require certain free radicals, because millions of chemical reactions take place each second in our cells and much of our biochemistry requires that electrons be transferred from molecule to molecule. Free radicals, since they tend to give and take electrons, often play an important role in these processes—and each cell in our bodies produces tens of thousands of them every day.

This situation is what some experts in the field have called "the oxygen paradox." As Jeffrey Blumberg, Ph.D., of the Human Nutrition Research Center on Aging at Tufts University, says, "We depend on oxygen—we must breathe. What's hard to understand is that oxygen has a dark side—that oxygen and free radicals are extraordinarily toxic to the body."[2]

Free Radicals and Other "Bad Guys"

The most common free radicals are built on oxygen molecules. Oxygen's molecular structure is especially suited for chemical reactions involving electron transfers. Dr. Pryor explains: "Oxygen is a strange molecule. When you have a molecule with an even number of electrons, the ground state is almost always one in which the electrons are paired up. In the ground state, oxygen has an even number of electrons, but two of them are unpaired. Quantum mechanics says you can only have two electrons in one orbital and they must have opposed spins. Oxygen's two unpaired electrons have the same spin, so they cannot go into the same orbital."[3]

Recall that a free radical is a molecule with an unpaired electron, looking for a mate. Oxygen molecules, with their two unpaired electrons, are twice as thirsty for electrons, making them highly reactive with other molecules. Oxygen itself can be harmful, and many processes in the body transform oxygen into a variety of other reactive molecules collectively referred to as *oxidants:* free radicals, oxy radicals, and reactive oxygen species (ROS).

Superoxide is often the first free radical formed and therefore is called the master oxygen radical. It consists of an oxygen molecule plus one electron. Superoxide is destructive itself; but it also easily converts into hydrogen peroxide and produces the hydroxyl radical.

Hydroxyl radicals are the most dangerous free radicals, and consist of equal parts of hydrogen and oxygen. Hydroxyl radicals are so reactive they last only .000000001 second; they will attack just about any other molecule they come into contact with, trying to donate their unpaired electron.

Hydrogen peroxide is a relatively long-lasting molecule that can pass through a cell membrane and harm the inside of the cell. When it reacts with superoxide or with "free" iron molecules, it forms the hydroxyl radical.

Lipid peroxy radicals are formed when oxygen attacks the fatty acids in cell membranes. During this lipid peroxidation, the fat molecules release more free radicals, initiating a deadly chain reaction across the membrane of the cell. This same process is what makes meat left out on your counter turn rancid.

Singlet oxygen is oxygen that has been "excited," which pairs up its two odd electrons and puts it into a "singlet state." Dr. Pryor points out that "this is the opposite of most molecules, which are even (paired) in the ground state, but unpair their electrons when you excite them." Singlet oxygen has an extremely short life—microseconds, and because it is formed mainly in the skin in response to untraviolet light, some scientists, including William Pryor, believe it isn't very important in biology, although it may cause skin cancer.[4]

The "Redox" Balance

When a molecule loses an electron, this process is called *oxidation;* when it gains an electron, the term *reduction* is used. As part of our normal metabolism, molecules are continually being oxidized and reduced so that a balance is maintained. Together, the oxidation–reduction processes that occur on a cellular level are called *redox reactions,* or the *redox potential.*

Within each of the trillions of our living cells occurs a rate of activity "so rapid as to challenge comprehension," writes Hari Sharma, M.D., author of *Freedom from Disease.* In his book, he tells us to "imagine an aerial view of the intense automobile and pedestrian traffic in New York City—speeded up millions of times. That's what life is like inside every cell of your body."[5]

Much of this action involves oxygen and its role in the cell's energy-creating system—a system not yet fully understood. Each cell has *mitochondria,* tiny energy generators that are packed with electron processors—100,000 in each one. Each processor in turn is composed of a sequence of enzymes that pass electrons down from one to the next. Down this *electron transport chain* flow electrons that have been stripped from glucose molecules, converting the energy into adenosine triphosphate (ATP), "like a waterfall turning a turbine to create electricity," according to Dr. Sharma.

At the end of the electron transport chain, an oxygen molecule accepts the electron, thus preventing the electrons from backing up in the chain. The final enzyme immediately combines the oxygen molecule with hydrogen, creating water, which is harmless. But during normal energy metabolism, a small percentage of electrons stray and are prematurely snatched from the chain by oxygen molecules. The extra electron turns oxygen molecules into superoxide molecules, which in turn produce other free radicals and reactive oxygen species. So, without oxygen to accept the electron at the end of the chain, we would not have this highly efficient energy system; neither would we have oxy radicals—the price we pay in exchange.

The other major natural and necessary source of free radicals is our immune system; immune cells produce free radicals to destroy bacteria and other invaders. White blood cells called neutrophils ingest the invaders, then take in huge amounts of oxygen in what's called a *respiratory burst*. These oxygen-rich cells then cook up a slew of oxy radicals and reactive oxygen species to kill the invaders. Macrophages—another type of white blood cell—arrive on the scene and in their own respiratory burst also subject the invader to free radical assault.

Without free radical oxidation, *aerobic* (oxygen-requiring) creatures like us wouldn't be able to blink, or think, or ride a bike, or pet a puppy, or read a book about antioxidants. We also couldn't fend off infection. Without redox balance, free radicals would spread out of control and damage so much tissue that we wouldn't be able to do anything. Under normal metabolic conditions, free radicals exist for incredibly short periods of time—fractions of a microsecond. They immediately become neutralized, or "mopped up," by components of our antioxidant defense system.

We have evolved these control mechanisms so that the harmful consequences to the cell (via runaway free radical chain reactions) remain small. During the ongoing actions and interactions that characterize human cellular metabolism, a continual tug-of-war takes place between the oxidation molecules and the antioxidants. Under normal circumstances these forces are equal enough to maintain a balance.

Stephen Levine, Ph.D., a free radical expert, author, and president of the Allergy Research Group in California, compares our normal metabolism to a burning log in a fireplace. We burn the wood to provide needed energy to maintain life, but this also creates stray sparks. Fortunately, we have a protective screen so that sparks from the fire don't stray far and start fires in our clothes or furniture. This "screen" is composed of our antioxidant defense system; the "sparks" are free radicals, which are a normal consequence of cellular metabolism, and represent certain inefficiencies in the burning process. The free radicals are potentially damaging if our screen is old or in disrepair, or if it has been overwhelmed by too many sparks created by exposure to harmful substances in our environment, emotional stress, or infection.

Our Defense System: Antioxidants to the Rescue

As we have seen, our living cells require oxygen to create energy and perform other functions, but paradoxically oxygen itself can be toxic to cells, particularly when it is converted to free radicals. Free radicals and an oxygen-based metabolism are part of our long evolutionary history, as are the biochemical defenses that the body has developed against their potential harmful effects. As one research team put it, "although free radicals are ubiquitous, they are by no means omnipotent."

The antioxidant defense system gives our bodies the ability to use oxygen during normal metabolism, and the ability to "quench" free radical by-products to avoid damage. Our normal cell chemistry is a never-ending process of oxygen damage and repair: one step forward, one step back. Our antioxidant defense system is made of a number of mechanisms, all of which aim to neutralize the radicals in some way. These strategies employ special enzymes that are produced in the body, as well as small quencher molecules created in the body and certain nutrients that we get from food or supplements. In the words of Richard Passwater, Ph.D., researcher and author of several books on nutrition and antioxidants, antioxidants "are compounds that do not generate free radicals during a reaction ... [they] combine readily with oxygen and neutralize oxygen radicals; the free radical chains are thus broken and other compounds and body compounds are [protected]."[6]

Enzymes are thought of as the "first line" of defense against radical oxidants; they work primarily from within the individual cells. Quencher molecules are the second line of defense; they operate primarily outside the cells. And radicals that slip past the first two lines are trapped by the last line of defense—those derived from nutrients. (Nutrients also play a role in the first line of defense since they are required for the enzymes themselves to function.)

ANTIOXIDANT ENZYMES

Enzyme systems that defuse free radicals are made by the cells according to instructions contained in the DNA. The major antioxidant enzymes are *superoxide dismutase (SOD), glutathione peroxidase (GP),* and *catalase*. Each plays a distinct role.

Superoxide dismutase is created solely to protect against superoxide, the most common free radical. SOD defuses the superoxide molecule by giving its extra electron a proton. It then adds a hydrogen atom, producing hydrogen peroxide (H_2O_2). Hydrogen peroxide itself is reactive, but less so than superoxide; it is also less harmful than the hydroxyl radical that superoxide would have created without SOD's intervention. Different forms of SOD are produced and used in different parts of the cell, and they require different metals (minerals) as *cofactors*. The SOD enzyme of the mitochondria, where most superoxide is formed, needs manganese. The SOD enzyme found in the cell plasma needs zinc and copper.

The *glutathione peroxidase* system is more complex. This enzyme continues the job begun by SOD—it transforms hydrogen peroxide by donating an electron. GP itself thus loses one electron, but this is replenished by another enzyme, *glutathione reductase*. Yet a third enzyme is needed to create glutathione from amino acids and selenium. The GP system also scavenges lipid peroxides by donating an electron. This enzyme system prevents other radicals, such as the dreaded hydroxyl radical, from being produced in several ways, and in so doing—as one expert puts it—"defuses an explosion of potential damage."

Catalase, it is now believed, plays a relatively minor role in antioxidant protection. It decomposes hydrogen peroxide into water and oxygen, but apparently only in tiny organelles (structures) within the cell called peroxisomes. This enzyme requires iron to function.

Without enzymes such as SOD, free radicals would eventually undergo *spontaneous dismutation,* a process during which the activated oxygen molecules react with themselves, thus quenching their mutual thirst for electrons. Through a series of steps, the molecules recombine (dismutate) and form harmless substances, such as stable oxygen molecules (O_2) and water (H_2O—hydrogen plus oxygen). This process, though spontaneous, moves very slowly, unless antioxidant enzymes are present to act as catalysts. Superoxide dismutase (SOD), for example, causes dismutation to proceed at a rate that is ten million times faster than when it is allowed to occur spontaneously.

Another defense mechanism involves repair. As one researcher describes it, "Enzymes snip out the bad sections of the DNA and replace them with good ones—sort of the analogy of the plumber replacing rusted sections of pipe with good ones."[7] According to Bruce Ames, a noted biochemist at the University of California at Berkeley, the average cell receives ten thousand daily "hits" from oxidized molecules—but almost every one of them is repaired.

QUENCHER MOLECULES

These molecules, produced by the body, donate electrons to neutralize free radicals. They include *uric acid,* which protects against superoxide, the hydroxyl radical, and lipid peroxy radicals. Test tube studies show that uric acid matches vitamin C in effectiveness against superoxide; researcher Bruce Ames speculates that this molecule helps counteract our inability to produce vitamin C in the body (see Chapter 3). Another quencher molecule is *ceruloplasmin,* a protein that scavenges superoxide, the hydroxyl radical, and singlet oxygen.

ANTIOXIDANT NUTRIENTS

Working closely with the antioxidant enzymes, antioxidants derived from nutrients act as "scavengers" that "mop up" reactive molecules and prevent destructive chain reactions. Compounds in this category include vitamin C (ascorbic acid), vitamin E (tocopherol), beta-carotene (provitamin A), vitamin A (retinol), and some amino acids.

Remember, there are five major oxidants: superoxide radicals, hydrogen peroxide, hydroxyl radicals, lipid peroxy radicals, and singlet oxygen. Enzymes are capable of dealing with only two: superoxide dismutase neutralizes superoxide, and glutathione peroxidase and catalase interact with hydrogen peroxide. This is where nutrients enter the picture.

Vitamin C provides protection against damage from superoxide and the hydroxyl radical. Vitamin E protects against singlet oxygen damage and polyunsaturated fatty acid (PUFA) lipid peroxy radicals. Beta-carotene quenches singlet oxygen molecules and PUFA radicals. Selenium protects against PUFA radicals. If the cell membranes do not have adequate levels of beta-carotene, vitamins C and E, or selenium, cells are more vulnerable to lipid oxidation.

All of these antioxidant enzymes, molecules, nutrients, and nutrient cofactors are important, and all work together as a highly efficient system. For example, when vitamin E interrupts a free radical chain reaction, it becomes a vitamin E radical; it is thought that vitamin E is regenerated from its radical form by vitamin C and glutathione. Therefore you need a sufficient amount of *both* vitamin E and C to control cell membrane damage. Jeffrey Bland, Ph.D., a nutrition and antioxidant specialist and director of HealthComm, a consulting firm, says, "These antioxidants work as buddies." He compares them to "a little molecular machine":

> Free radicals are quenched in a sequential series of steps. My analogy would be a Pachinko game—the ball comes in the top but it touches a lot of little things on the way down before it falls out the bottom. That's what free radical chemistry does— they are sequentially detoxified by a series of little steps and they gradually get less and less harmful with each step.[8]

The Bad News

This system is designed to be highly efficient and effective under normal circumstances. However, many scientists argue that modern conditions are far from "normal." We are subject to an unprecedented amount of environmental and perhaps psychological stresses that increase the production of free radicals or disable our antioxidant defenses, or both. This translates into an increase in *oxidative stress* and causes an imbalance.

In the redox tug-of-war, if the oxidation molecules outweigh the antioxidants, the equilibrium is lost. As the balance of power shifts toward excessive oxidation, a kind of structural meltdown spreads throughout nearby molecules. Thus begins the chain reaction of proliferating free radicals leading to a cascade of damaged molecules, and perhaps to damaged cells, tissues, and organs. In Chapter 2 we take a look at what free radical researchers believe occurs when free radical reactions spread out of control, and why. But first, it is important to understand which factors can shift the redox balance in the first place.

Contributors to Oxidative Stress

In addition to the oxidation required to maintain basic metabolism, our bodies produce higher levels of free radicals and other oxidants during exercise; after physical trauma such as burns; after strokes, heart attacks, and injuries; and during infections. Chronic emotional stress may also produce excess free radicals since it raises the level of certain hormones (epinephrine and norepinephrine), which tend to oxidize easily and become free radicals. Aging itself seems to slow down the production and function of the various antioxidant mechanisms, and thus throw off the redox balance. Dr. Bland explains:

> There's a whole series of both external and internal agents that can initiate an increase of reactive oxygen species in the body for which the level of demand on antioxidants is greater. Certainly ionizing radiation—cosmic and x-radiation—[creates free radicals]. And to some degree photodynamic action is related to the production of singlet oxygen through ultraviolet

radiation. We know that rancid food products contain free radical catalysts like lipid peroxides; we know that cigarette smoke, drugs, and alcohol and other chemicals contain them too. And we know that the body under its own processes produces oxidants.[9]

ENVIRONMENTAL POLLUTION

We are exposed to an astonishing variety of chemical pollutants through our air, water, and food. Many are bad for our health, but it isn't always clear how or why, although it may be because they contain or catalyze the release of free radicals in our systems. There are about 70,000 synthetic chemicals on the market, half of which are in common use. Only 800 have been tested to see if they produce cancer, let alone cause oxidation.

Stephen Levine has studied environmental free radicals and has published widely on the subject. He believes:

> There are strong experimental indications that in many cases the damaging effects are not due to the original compound itself, but to an oxidized version of it. When our body encounters such compounds, either through the air, water, or food, our body detoxifies them, and converts them to reactive molecules and free radicals, as an intermediate step. These intermediates may be more damaging than the original ("parent") chemical.[10]

Many environmental poisons such as pesticides, industrial chemicals, and drugs are treated similarly by the body. During the detoxification process, they are sometimes broken down, creating hydrogen peroxide, superoxide, or a special type of radical that, in effect, works like a free radical factory. During this process, called *redox recycling,* the radical steals electrons—probably from the electron transport chain—and passes them on to oxygen, creating a continuous supply of new oxy radicals.

Smog is a rich source of oxidants. According to Levine, 22 compounds are found in smog that promote oxidation; these include ozone, nitrogen oxides, and carbon monoxide. Much outdoor air pollution is produced by transportation vehicles burning fossil fuel. Cars contribute more pollution than any other form of transportation. We've known for decades that these pollutants, produced by cars, trucks, buses, and industries, are harmful to our lungs. Air pollution is known to be the leading cause of lung diseases such as emphysema, bronchitis, and asthma. Ozone—a molecule composed of three oxygen atoms—is believed to be the most toxic component of air pollution, and has been the most studied. At ground level, ozone is formed when sunlight interacts with nitrogen dioxide and unburned hydrocarbons from fuel.

More than 100 million Americans are exposed to levels of ozone higher than the maximum safe level currently set by the U.S. Environmental Protection Agency. This is particularly troublesome because the evidence shows that ozone's adverse health effects on the respiratory tract occur within the current range of exposure levels of many Americans. Daniel Menzel, Ph.D., a free radical researcher at the University of California at Irvine, has specialized in studying air pollution and lung disease. In an article written in 1992 he points out that efforts to reduce car and truck emissions have thus far not been able to reduce nitrogen dioxide to a safe level in most major cities.

Menzel writes: "Animal studies have shown that ozone and nitrogen dioxide are the two most toxic of the air pollutants."[11] In a variety of species, including rats and primates, the experimental animals developed diseases similar to human bronchitis when exposed to nitrogen dioxide, and emphysema when exposed to ozone. He notes that the diseases occurred after a near lifetime exposure at levels that were near those typical of air pollution. This toxicity correlates well with the observation that in both animals and humans, exposure to ozone and nitrogen dioxide increases lung permeability or causes inflammation. Patients with preexisting asthma are particularly sensitive. Moreover, once lung damage is evident anatomically, it is usually irreversible, even when exposure to these pollutants is stopped.

Children who live in highly polluted areas have been shown to experience lung damage, including decreased lung development. A year after the record-high smog levels of 1988, researchers in Los Angeles studied the lungs of 100 young people who had died in accidents or from other non-health-related causes. They found that 80 of them had lung damage, and in 27, the damage was severe. Menzel finds these data "alarming." As he puts it: "The lungs of these children fail to keep up with the growth of their bodies."[12] Like many researchers, he believes that we should act early to prevent exposed children from getting respiratory disease as adults, just as we use fluoride to protect against tooth decay.

Dr. Levine writes:

No one in the field of photochemical oxidants has gone to the level of stating that the toxicity of smog is due to free radicals, that the reactive metabolites and not the parent compounds are toxic. However, that seems to be the inevitable conclusion: from cancer and free radical research we do see plenty of hard data that the radical species are the toxic molecules.[13]

Dr. Menzel believes that "although the evidence for oxidative stress [from] air pollution in the human lung is fragmentary, the hypothesis that oxidative stress is an important, if not the sole, mechanism of toxicity of oxidizing air pollutants and tobacco smoke is compelling and growing."[14]

Likewise, the toxicity of heavy metal contaminants—lead, mercury, cadmium—found in water, food, and air may be due to their ability to initiate free radicals or otherwise upset the normal redox balance. Chlorine in our water supply reacts with organic matter in groundwater (for example, from plant debris) to create chlorinated hydrocarbons, which are radicals. Chloride compounds, used in the manufacturing of Saran Wrap and many other plastic products, are thought to be found throughout the United States in drinking water; once metabolized some produce free radicals.

Inhaled pollutants are of particular concern because they are taken into the lungs, where the alveoli (air sacs) are composed of very thin, delicate tissue, making the lung itself vulnerable to oxidative damage. In addition, whereas ingested pollutants first go to the liver for detoxification before they enter the general blood circulation, inhaled pollutants enter the blood directly, and therefore have access to all the organs before they are detoxified.

Cigarette smoke is a major source of oxidants and subjects the lungs and other organs to oxidative stress. "Cigarette smoke is probably one of the most effective ways to deliver very potent free radicals to your lungs. I can't think of a better way to do it,"[15] says Blumberg, the researcher from Tufts University. It is the primary cause of lung cancer and emphysema and is implicated in many other diseases and conditions in both smokers and those who are subjected to second-hand smoke. "Every puff of a cigarette has literally millions of free radicals," says Adrianne Bendich, Ph.D., a clinical research scientist at Hoffmann-La Roche, a leading manufacturing of antioxdant supplements. "A cigarette smoker has to consume 250 mg of vitamin C a day to reach the same blood levels as a nonsmoker achieves with 60 mg per day because vitamin C is used mopping up the free radicals. Vitamin E is lower in smokers, and so is beta-carotene."[16] As the body uses up antioxidant nutrients to neutralize oxidants from the smoke, the resulting imbalance in the redox potential could lead to an increased susceptibility to tissue damage and disease such as emphysema or cancer.

Several studies have shown that smokers have high levels of oxidants outside their cells; and that the more they have of these extracellular oxidants, the more likely they are to have lung disease. It is unlikely that this excess of free radicals is a result rather than a cause of lung disease, since a study of animals who were exposed to cigarette smoke for only 15 weeks showed increased levels of free radicals. Levine writes, "With cigarette smoke being such a concentrated source of free radical oxidant compounds, smoking is likely to be a major source of oxidative stress both to the lungs and other organs which become exposed to its constituents by way of circulation."[17]

Indoor air. Indoor air may be far more polluted than outdoor air, in part because of the materials used to build, heat, and furnish homes and offices, and in part because the energy-saving design of new buildings makes them so airtight that airborne pollutants become trapped and concentrated. In 1983 the research firm of Small and Associates evaluated indoor air pollution for the Canadian government. They found that cigarette smoke is the primary indoor air pollutant and source of free radicals for smokers and nonsmokers. Next is radon, a radioactive gas emitted by rocks and soil that accumulates in buildings. Then comes ozone, generated by many types of equipment, such as ultraviolet (UV) lamps and copying machines.

Formaldehyde, released (outgassed) by certain types of insulation and pressed wood furniture, is also an oxidant and acknowledged carcinogen. Gas-powered space heaters and cooking stoves give off nitrogen oxides and therefore are an additional source of indoor pollution; children who live in homes with gas cooking stoves tend to have a higher-than-average number of upper respiratory infections. Although, as Menzel is careful to explain, "these results are controversial inasmuch as tobacco smoking in the home also increases the upper respiratory infection rate . . . the controversy may be resolved when one considers that tobacco smoke contains large amounts of nitrogen oxides, which are converted to nitrogen dioxide."[18]

Asbestos fibers provide still another free-radical-related mechanism for trouble. They are believed to lead to cancer because the body unwittingly exposes itself to free radicals. As macrophages try to gobble up the impossibly long asbestos fibers lodged in the lungs, they create free radicals in an attempt to dissolve the fibers. Lung cells, under the onslaught, can mutate and become cancerous.

ALCOHOL AND OTHER DRUGS
Although some studies show that drinking alocholic beverages in moderation may actually have health benefits, particularly in relation to heart disease, alcohol also has its down side, especially if consumed in excessive amounts. When alcohol is metabolized in the body, free radicals form, damaging the body's tissues.

Chronic excess consumption of alcohol leads to cirrhosis of the liver, which may well be due to free radical mechanisms. When the blood of alcoholics was tested, researchers found elevated levels of a substance associated with free radical activity. In addition, antioxidants have been found to be useful in the prevention of alcohol-induced changes in fatty acids, suggesting that free radicals are involved in the process. Finally, prolonged drinking of alcohol also reduces the levels of protective nutrient antioxidants in liver cells and in the blood.

Certain common prescription and over-the-counter medications—including anti-inflammatories such as acetaminophen (Tylenol), anticonvulsant drugs such as phenytoin (Dilantin) and phenobarbital, and many broad-spectrum antibiotics—form free radicals, which may account for their side effects. The mechanism through which such drugs exact their oxidative toll is likely to be similar to that which occurs with environmental pollutants. As a first step toward elimination by the body, these external substances "are metabolized in the liver, and this produces free radicals as by-products," explains Adrianne Bendich.[19] These oxidants, however, cause damage before they can be eliminated. Cancer chemotherapy drugs such as adriamycin kill cancer cells through free radical oxidation. They kill normal cells by oxidation, too. The major toxic side effect of adriamycin is to the heart tissue; vitamin E, an antioxidant, has been shown to minimize this damage.

RADIATION

The recent wave of free radical research grew out of experiments with high-energy radiation, which gives rise to potent reactive molecules. Some molecules become "excited" as they absorb radiant energy. In this excited state, their electrons get shifted and this in turn transforms them into eager free radicals. Oxygen molecules are particularly vulnerable to light—including ultraviolet rays from the sun—and are easily excited when these rays hit them. Likewise, water molecules are sensitive to ionizing radiation such as X rays and gamma rays. It is believed that this process accounts for the damaging effects of radiation on the DNA and proteins in living things. Damage to DNA in turn can lead to genetic mutations and cancer.

Adrianne Bendich says,

> Sunlight generates singlet oxygen, which generates free radicals. We're not just talking skin cancer—singlet oxygen generates free radicals in the skin, but they circulate throughout the body. As a group, skin cancer patients have a higher rate for many other cancers, and there's a very strong UV compo nent in melanoma.[20]

Our species has evolved to survive in an environment that contains "background" radiation from rocks, the sun, and outer space. But the level of radiation to which we are exposed is rising due to a number of factors. These include a depleted ozone layer, which allows more ultraviolet rays to reach us; exposure to medical and dental X rays; the release of radioactivity into the environment by nuclear energy and nuclear weapons; and frequent airplane travel, which exposes us to atmospheric radiation.

DIET

Each cell of the body uses oxygen to create energy from nutrients. During this process, free radical oxygen molecules containing unpaired electrons are released. A diet that is high in fat can increase this free radical formation because oxidation occurs more readily in fat molecules than in carbohydrate or protein molecules. Polyunsaturated fats are more prone to oxidation than monounsaturated or saturated fats. Animal experiments show that diets high in polyunsaturated fats accelerate the free radical reactions in body tissues and enhance carcinogenesis.

In addition, diets high in animal fat are more likely to contain chemicals that form free radicals because these substances accumulate from the environment and are stored in the fat cells of the animal's body. Diets that contain large amounts of rancid (oxidized) fats increase free radical levels in the body. Usually antioxidants in the mucosal lining of the intestine make short shrift of small amounts of rancid oils, but this mechanism can become overtaxed, allowing free radicals to enter the bloodstream and attack other tissues. In particular, cooking fats at high temperatures—such as frying foods in hot oil—can produce large amounts of free radicals.

In addition, diets that are low in foods containing antioxidant nutrients (mainly fresh fruits and vegetables) may contribute to radical damage because they offer little support to our free radical defense system. As your mother said, eating vegetables is good for you—but now we know why. Processed foods such as white flour and sugars are by definition depleted of the vitamins and minerals contained in whole fresh foods. Caffeine in the diet (contained in coffee, tea, colas, and chocolate, but also found in some medications) provides a temporary lift, but can increase free radical formation.

Stephen Levine wrote in *The Journal of Orthomolecular Psychiatry:*

With the rapidly accelerating rate of growth of modern technology has come a proliferation of chemicals totally unprecedented in human evolution. There are now thousands of chemicals dispersed in the ecosphere; their molecular structures are diverse, and their effects upon biological systems are bound to be varied. Though these chemicals . . . may differ in their physiochemical characteristics and in their mode of entry to the body . . . [and] their biological effects will inevitably require thousands of toxicologists millions of hours to unravel, rest assured that the overriding theme of their toxicity is by some expression of oxidative stress to our bodies.[21]

Many free radical researchers believe that the more environmental, dietary, and quite possibly psychological stress factors in your life, the greater the oxidative stress on your body. Your antioxidant defense system is taxed beyond its normal, natural capabilities. Unless the stress is reduced and the antioxidant nutrients replenished, your body is at risk for extensive free radical damage and a wide range of diseases and disorders.

TWO

Free Radical Overload:

TIPPING THE BALANCE TOWARD DISEASE

■

When the body is overloaded with free radicals, or the anti-oxidant defense system has become weakened, the radicals are created faster than the body can handle them. This overload first leads to *oxidative stress*. Evidence has been accumulating for decades supporting the theory that oxidative stress is a factor in aging and, according to some researchers, may lead to more than 60 degenerative diseases such as cancer, heart disease, cataracts, and immune and neurological diseases. If they are right, future research may provide us with ways to prevent or slow down these conditions—and perhaps even reverse them, especially in their earliest stages.

How the Body Responds

Both human and animal studies show that when oxidative stress increases, the boy is designed to respond to the situation by increasing the amount of antioxidant enzymes produced. The increase in the amount of antioxidants naturally increases their activity. For example, when the lungs of experimental animals were exposed to ozone, levels of two antioxidant enzymes, glutathione peroxidase and superoxide dismutase, became more active. The antioxidant system rises to the occasion, oxidant damage is minimized, and the lung cell membranes are protected.

But what if the oxidative stress occurs again before the body is able to replenish its stores of antioxidants? What happens when the body is chronically exposed to an excess of free radicals from the factors discussed in Chapter 1? It appears that damage first occurs to the molecules of individual cells; when damage accumulates and cells die or are unable to function, extensive tissue damage may result; if the process still goes unchecked, it results in organ damage and disease.

CELL DAMAGE

It appears that free radicals, using varied and complex mechanisms, can attack any component of the cell: fat, protein, and carbohydrate molecules, cell membranes, genetic material (DNA), and biochemical compounds needed to keep the body running smoothly. Researchers are still searching for answers to the question of exactly which parts of the cell are most vulnerable to oxidative damage.

The cell membranes, thin walls that surround the outer cell and the structures within it, seem most susceptible. The damage they undergo has been studied most and is the best understood. Most of the electron transfers in cells occur in the membranes. They are rich in fat molecules (fatty acids, or *lipids*). Any fat—saturated fatty acids, monounsaturated fatty acids, cholesterol, or unsaturated fatty acids—can be oxidized and turned rancid. But free radicals are particularly attracted to polyunsaturated fatty acids (PUFAs) because of their molecular structure, which has a dense concentration of electrons. Cell membranes that are highest in this form of fatty acid are especially at risk. What's more, although cell membranes also contain protein molecules, these are relatively sparsely distributed among the fat molecules. The result is a smooth, uninterrupted lipid "lake" for free radicals to propagate across. Unless stopped in time by antioxidants, the structure of the membrane can become so corroded that the cell wall collapses and the cell dies.

Protein molecules are also vulnerable to oxidation, from nearby lipid free radicals and their by-products as well as from other radicals. Although low in population compared with fat molecules, proteins have a potent presence in cell membranes: they function as receptors, antigens, and enzymes that allow for the transport of substances into and out of the cell. Once damaged, the cell membrane can no longer function as effectively.

When either its fats or its proteins are damaged, according to researcher Richard Passwater, "the membrane does not properly function to take nutrients into the cell and to remove waste products, and so the cell cannot reproduce itself and dies due to starvation or drowning in waste products."[1] Oxidation can depress the activity of phagocytes—cells that engulf and digest microorganisms, harmful cells, and other foreign invaders—and this creates an immune system deficiency. Free radicals can also damage the mitochondrial walls inside the cell, hampering the cell's ability to create energy. Radicals can also injure cell structures called lysosomes, which digest certain bacteria, particles, and cellular debris. As a result, the enzymes in the lysosomes leak out and inadvertently digest needed parts of the cell. Again, we have cell death.

In addition, free radicals damage DNA. Damaged DNA cannot make the enzymes required for metabolic processes. Free-radical-induced mutations in the DNA can also lead to cancer and other diseases. According to Anthony Diplock, a free radical researcher at the University of London, "There is ample evidence that in vitro the presence of a free radical [generator] . . . in close proximity to DNA will result in extensive damage to the DNA structure."[2] One further mechanism of damage occurs when free radicals fuse protein together in a process called *cross-linking*—in effect, welding molecules together—preventing them from frunctioning normally. This can eventually lead to cell death, and is how some drugs used in cancer chemotherapy kill cancer cells—and some normal cells, too, as an unfortunate side effect.

Jeffrey Bland, Ph.D., cautions against labeling free radicals as bad per se and labeling things that trap free radicals as "good." He reminds us that cholesterol was labeled "bad," although it is essential for proper health at certain levels, and that at controlled levels, free radicals actually participate in a variety of important metabolic functions. "The real question to me is, what is the *redox potential* of the body because that's how we control metabolically the exposure to both the boon and bane of oxygen," Bland says.[3] "If the redox potential in the cells is well controlled, the person is in homeostasis, the person has a high organ reserve and is healthy." He goes on to explain that

under conditions of disease, it is known that the redox potential of the body is disturbed. At that point the processes start to wind down and we get more production of the oxidant molecules which are not trapped or quenched effectively and then engage in chain reaction damage to the body. That's why people in a hospital emergency room or critical care center can go south healthwise very quickly. They might be doing okay and then in the next hour look like they're going into full organ shutdown. These reactions occur geometrically and if they're not trapped they can overwhelm the physiology very rapidly.[4]

FREE-RADICAL-RELATED DISEASES

A variety of serious and not-so-serious diseases and conditions have been blamed on free radicals, based on the theory that cell damage accumulates and progresses to tissue damage and then organ damage. Until recently, much of this evidence has come from studies of cells or from animal studies, or else has been inferred from epidemiological studies that examine what people were exposed to or the level of antioxidants in their diets. In many instances, the connection between free radicals and disease remains circumstantial or theoretical, but the data is incriminating enough to convince many responsible researchers that free radicals could play a significant role in many disease processes that have puzzled us for centuries.

Bland says, "It is clearly obvious to most people in the field . . . that a variety of inflammatory-related conditions which are chronic in nature and lead to increasing morbidity and premature mortality, all have their association with free radical oxidant damage." He includes in this category coronary artery disease, certain forms of cancer, certain forms of arthritis, gastrointestinal inflammatory diseases, and maybe even neurological dysfunctions that are associated with myelin destruction and central nervous system damage such as Alzheimer's disease, multiple sclerosis, and the later-stage neurological effects of diabetes.[5]

AGING AND LIFE SPAN

In spite of decades of intense study, scientists are not sure what causes aging—or even exactly what aging is. However, there is widespread agreement that free radicals play a role. Huber R. Warner of the National Institute on Aging wrote in 1993: "Aging is a complex set of interactions between environmental insults and genetically defined factors. . . . I believe that oxidative damage is a major component of these environmental insults."[6]

In presenting this view, Warner discusses research studies that help provide a picture of the currently known relationships between free radicals and longevity. For example, he concludes that while it is difficult to establish "unequivocal support for the free radical theory of aging," he was able to find a number of positive correlations. The evidence suggests that the more free radicals produced in the body, the shorter the life span; a synthetic antioxidant (phenylnitrone) might slow aging; very low-calorie diets delay age-related changes and "affect a wide variety of processes which may be related to oxidative damage"; and when the level of antioxidant production is genetically altered to increase, life spans also increase.

Many of the processes linked with free radical damage are degenerative in nature, and have been associated with abnormal, accelerated aging and its telltale signs of sagging, wrinkled, age-spotted skin; failing memory and concentration; flagging energy and lack of stamina; stiff joints; and a sluggish, disorganized immune system. Our risk of cancer, heart disease, arthritis, and Alzheimer's disease and our susceptibility to infection rises with each birthday, and all of these have been linked with free radical damage as well.

Perhaps a certain amount of wear and tear is an inevitable part of living, just as our cars wear out and stop running. But according to some free radical theorists, excess free radicals cause our body parts to "rust" or wear out faster than they have to. If we could stem the tide of damage, our arteries, joints and ligaments, lungs, kidneys, heart, brain, eyes, and skin would all function better longer—and we might look younger too.

Oxidation of fats in our cell membranes may play a major role in aging. The *mitochondria* (the internal powerhouses of the cells) in particular may become progressively "worn down"; this is a suspected mechanism in the onset of age-related disorders including Parkinson's disease and adult-onset diabetes. Many researchers believe that the mitochondrial membrane may be the Achilles' heel of an aging cell. As we age, damaged components of the cell build up. This accumulation of useless molecules is called *lipofuscin*. It appears as yellowish or brownish spots and globs (hence the term *age pigment*) in our bodies, particularly the heart, brain, and liver. The age spots that appear on our skin are in part composed of lipofuscin.

In his booklet *The Antioxidants,* free radical researcher Richard Passwater, Ph.D., describes aging as "the process that reduces the number of healthy cells in the body," and says that "the most striking factor in the aging process is the body's loss of reserve due to the decreasing amount of cells in each organ."[7] Since free radical reactions result in the loss of active cells, the cumulative effect of billions of reactions causes the body to lose its reserve.

Several researchers have been able to extend the average life span of animals with single antioxidant nutrients. For example, Passwater's experiments with synergistic combinations of nutrients extended the average life span of animals by 20 to 30 percent, and their maximum life span by 5 to 10 percent.[8]

Bland believes controlling free radical damage won't likely extend our maximum life span, but can help us extend the number of years we remain healthy. He says,

Certainly it can facilitate improvements in what we call the rate of biological aging. The concept of senescence and death is a very complex process that goes beyond daily metabolic activities. We must look at larger scale circadian changes that occur in the hormonal and immunological system, that are in part related to messages that are encoded in our genes. There's a long-standing debate whether we have a "death hormone" that is produced [by our bodies, or] whether we have damage to the DNA which accumulates and ultimately results in poor metabolic performance because the daughter cells aren't capable of performing as their parents. So what we're really saying on the basis of organ reserve, is that protection against accelerated radical processes is certainly desirable, and I do believe that following that line of research will open up all sorts of ways that we have previously not acknowledged for extending one's functional capabilities.[9]

ATHEROSCLEROSIS AND HEART DISEASE

Atherosclerosis is the accumulation of plaque on the inside walls of blood vessels. The plaque deposits are a waxy cheeselike substance, and this fibrous tissue gradually causes the arteries to narrow. Deposits occur in any of the large and medium-sized arteries, but particularly in the coronary arteries that go to the heart and the cerebral arteries that supply the brain. (Arteriosclerosis, which is often confused with atherosclerosis, consists of changes in the walls of the arteries that lead them to become hard and thick from calcium deposits and the effects of chronic high blood pressure.) Atherosclerosis is involved in about half of all death and illness in the United States. Narrowed arteries are susceptible to blockage from blood clots; this can cause heart attack (when a coronary artery is blocked) or stroke (when a cerebral artery is affected). Narrow arteries may also become so constricted that angina (chest pains) or intermittent claudication (leg pain) occurs.

A large body of evidence indicates that high cholesterol

levels do not by themselves cause arteries to become clogged. It is now thought that atherosclerosis is initiated by free radicals, which attack the lipids in the cells of the lining of the arteries. They also oxidize the low-density lipoproteins (the LDLs, or "bad" form of cholesterol), turning them into free radicals that injure the lining cells of the vessel wall. The damage attracts immune cells (neutrophils and monocytes) to the site; these release more free radicals and create more cellular damage. The monocytes then mature into macrophages and stuff themselves with circulating oxidized LDL; because of their foamy appearance they are known as foam cells. Fatty streaks begin to accumulate on the artery walls, and platelets pile up in the debris and cause blood to clot. The resulting deposits build up, causing atherosclerosis.

Several other findings support the theory that free radicals play a role in atherosclerosis. When lesions are examined microscopically, we find that they contain oxidized fat, and the amount of oxidation corresponds to the severity of the deposit. People with diagnosed heart disease and with diabetes and chronic smokers all have high levels of free radical products circulating in their plasma. Cigarette smoking is correlated with atherosclerosis; the death rate from coronary heart disease is 70 percent higher for smokers than for nonsmokers.

Iron and other metals such as copper react with oxygen, and this may in part explain why premenopausal women are at lower risk for heart disease than men. Iron is normally locked up tight by hemoglobin in red blood cells or firmly attached to proteins that transport it to where it is needed. However, under certain conditions it can become detached and free to cause radical mayhem. Some scientists believe that our iron-fortified foods and iron supplements are creating excessively high stores of iron, and overtaxing our body's ability to handle it. Women who menstruate rid their bodies of excess iron, lowering the risk of oxidation, and presumably atherosclerosis and heart attack.

A researcher at New York University, Dr. Harry Demopoulos, theorizes that atherosclerosis affects every organ of the body—not just the heart and brain. As it restricts blood flow to cells, tissues, and organs, the lack of oxygen and nutrients literally starves them and causes them gradually to waste away. The major organs shrink as we age: heart, brain, bones, liver, genitals, all shrivel, perhaps in part due to free radical damage to the feeder arteries.

An antioxidant drug called probucol has been shown to slow the progression of atherosclerosis in animals, but the drug has unwanted side effects. Nutritional antioxidants have also shown great potential in slowing atherosclerosis, without side effects, in test tube experiments as well as in animals and humans. As you'll see in the next chapter on antioxidant vitamins, studies show that high levels of vitamin E may reduce the risk of heart disease in men and women by 40 percent; high levels of vitamin C reduce death from heart disease and other causes in men by 40 percent; and beta-carotene supplements can cut the risk of heart attack in half among men with a history of cardiovascular disease. In addition, wine appears to contain a potent antioxidant that blocks LDL oxidative damage. This finding may help explain what has been dubbed "the French paradox"—that the French eat foods high in saturated fat and cholesterol, but suffer a fraction of the lethal heart disease of people in the United States. However, the French also eat more fruits and vegetables than we do, and this needs to be considered along with the antioxidant effects of red wine.

CANCER

Cancer is diagnosed in more than one million people in the United States each year; half of these eventually will die of the disease. Cancer is believed to arise from a combination of external factors and a hereditary predisposition. Current thinking is that cancer is a multistep process by which a normal cell becomes changed, loses its normal identity and structure (differentiation), and multiplies out of control. The cell's DNA receives a number of injuries or "hits" over the course of time, and each hit nudges it one step closer to full-fledged cancer. The hits may be through viruses, radiation, or chemicals.

In line with this theory is the belief that cancer is multi-factorial—usually we can't pin it on any *one* factor or type of "hit." For example, even people who inherit a defective gene for a type of cancer will not get that cancer unless they get another "hit" from the environment. It is thought that cancers that are virus-related follow the same rules: the virus may introduce defective genes into the cell, but that is just the first step toward carcinogenesis. Cancer risk increases with age, and this is in part because the accumulation of hits increases in proportion to age.

After *initiation,* other factors serve to promote the growth of mutated cells. This process can occur quite slowly in humans. Finally, during the phase of *progression,* the cell becomes malignant (cancerous).

Free radicals are implicated in the development of cancer directly, by their ability to damage the DNA in the cell nucleus, and by weakening the immune system, which normally destroys cancer cells or prevents them from reproducing. A carcinogen usually undergoes a transformation inside the body—it is metabolized or detoxified and becomes a metabolite, many of which are free radicals. These may react with the nucleus of the cell, damaging the DNA. In a strong antioxidant defense system, the free radical is neutralized before it can damage DNA, or the damage is detected and repaired. But if not, the cell with abnormal DNA replicates and so begins the process of cancer.

Strong evidence that free radical damage is involved in the development of cancer comes from the work of Donald C. Malins, Ph.D., at the Pacific Northwest Research Foundation in Washington. In 1993, Malins and researchers at the University of Washington published the results of their breakthrough study on free radicals and breast cancer.[10] Dr. Malins had previously used sophisticated new technology to identify DNA that had been altered by free radicals in the liver tumors of fish from Puget Sound. He then moved on to the study of human tissue. Malins describes his accomplishment:

> There was a lot of work in the lab on free radicals in rats and mice, and even suggesting that this was a problem with people. But no one had ever demonstrated the presence of and structurally elucidated these lesions in any tissues before—that's what was the breakthrough. Once we had the capability of looking at human tissues it opened up a vast area for seeing what was actually happening to DNA in living systems.[11]

Dr. Malins decided to focus on breast cancer and in a small preliminary study was able to identify specific alterations in the DNA of breast cancer tumors. He next conducted a controlled study using discarded tissue from healthy breasts that had been surgically reduced in size; this he compared with breast tissue removed from women with cancerous breasts. Malins continues:

> We ultimately were able to develop 22 statistical models to project the causation of the lesion formations. We discovered

that a pivotal event in the etiology of breast cancer was a shift in the redox potential of the breast towards increased oxidative status, which then stressed the DNA, presumably at a rate faster than it could be repaired. As a result, you have damaged DNA.[12]

The team found that the DNA changes were present not only in the tumor itself, but throughout the whole breast, "even in the tissue surrounding the tumor that appeared microscopically normal," according to Malins. This explains why surgically removing the tumor still leaves the woman at risk of a second tumor erupting at a later date. This study not only provides important insight as to how breast cancer develops, but also offers a potential means of predicting cancer development before cancer cells are formed, as well as suggests that antioxidants may reverse the process of initiation and prevent cancer on a cellular level. (These implications are discussed in Chapter 7: The Future of Antioxidants.)

Many of the antioxidant nutrients have been associated with a lower risk of cancer, supporting the idea that free radicals play a role in carcinogenesis. It is thought that antioxidants help prevent hits from occurring and accumulating, and that they also stimulate the immune system. For example, there is much evidence that selenium prevents cancer in animals; and strong epidemiological evidence that lower than normal levels of selenium are correlated with some kinds of cancer. The protective effect of selenium in cancer may be that of an antioxidant. Cancer researchers are interested in vitamin C and beta-carotene as protective agents because a substantial body of evidence shows that the incidence of cancer is lower in populations that eat large amounts of leafy green vegetables or fruit, which are good sources of these nutrients. As you'll see in the following chapter, in laboratory tests, vitamin C has been shown to act as a powerful suppressor of carcinogen formation. And two recent studies that measured the level of beta-carotene in the blood of a total of over 1,200 men showed a strong correlation between high levels of this antioxidant and lower incidence of cancer, especially lung cancer, even in smokers. In addition, many known animal and human carcinogens are oxidants, suggesting that oxidation is the mechanism by which they cause disease.

Interestingly, free radical oxidation is also the mechanism by which cancer chemotherapy drugs disable and kill cancer cells. The problem with these drugs is how not to kill the normal cells as well. There are several studies that show that adding antioxidant therapy to chemotherapy (and radiation treatments) reduces harmful side effects and improves the effectiveness of the cancer treatment.

IMMUNE DISORDERS

Our immune system has two main functions—to disarm foreign invaders such as microbes and to repair or dispose of damaged or worn out cells and tissues. It also is involved in the chemical communication among cells. The immune system and antioxidant system are interdependent. The same nutrients that act as antioxidants (beta-carotene, vitamins C and E, zinc, and selenium) are also needed for immune function. It seems highly probable that their antioxidant ability is the mechanism by which they improve and maintain immune function.

As explained earlier, the immune system uses free radicals to kill harmful bacteria. But true to their good news/bad news character, excess radicals can impair immune functioning. For example, when a cell membrane is damaged, so is its ability to communicate with the immune system, which depends on receptor cells for certain substances such as interleukins and immunoglobulins. At the cellular level, oxidation in this way can deactivate the immune system. Or the immune system may recognize an altered cell protein as something foreign and try to destroy it (autoimmunity.) In this way as well, oxidation alters normal immune response.

Both acute high-level and chronic low-level exposure to oxidant chemicals can impair the immune system. Lungs are particularly vulnerable: acute exposure causes reactions that resemble asthma—constricted breathing passages and difficulty breathing. The classic respiratory allergic reaction, sparked by airborne fungal, grass, or other plant allergens, results from a complex chain of events that begins with the oxidation of lipids in membranes of the lung.

The impact of free radicals on immune function may go far beyond the classic "allergic" reaction and cause our immune defenses to backfire. On the cellular level, our immune defenses react to a threat with a burst of metabolic activity, which increases the consumption of oxygen, especially by phagocytic cells, which create free radicals to destroy microbes within the cell. Under normal conditions, extensive free radical damage is believed to be avoided because the phagocytes engulf the microbes and so most of the toxic free radicals remain inside the cell and are directed only at microbes; antioxidants are able to neutralize any stray free radicals that are released outside the cell.

However, chronic or severe exposure to toxic substances leads to chronic or severe inflammation. This can eventually overwhelm the antioxidant system and inflict damage on bystander proteins and cells in the lungs, for example, ultimately leading to pulmonary fibrosis (scarring of the lung), emphysema, and cancer.

Adrianne Bendich, a specialist in vitamins and immune function, says that when the immune system is challenged,

> you need some free radicals and inflammatory products to be formed at the proper level and in the proper place. With bacteria and viruses, the killing process occurs in a special compartment within the cell so that the other parts of the cell are not exposed. But if there is an overproduction of free radicals, these immune cells overproduce inflammatory products. They can spew them out into the surrounding area, allowing these products to damage normal cells.[13]

Bendich compares the scenario to a speeding car. "If you drive a car at 45 miles per hour in a 45-mile-per-hour zone, it's okay, but if you're in a 20-mile-per-hour zone, you're in trouble."[14]

In his review article on antioxidants and lung disease, Daniel Menzel explains that oxidation of unsaturated fatty acids by either ozone or nitrogen dioxide produces substances called fatty aldehydes that act as inflammatory signals.[15] The incessant broadcast of such a signal, due to chronic exposure to air pollution or cigarette smoke, could be responsible for summoning inflammatory cells to the lungs. The reason antioxidant vitamins protect the body may be due in part to their ability to prevent inflammation, by blocking the production of the oxidative stress signal molecules. A study published in 1990 found that exposure to urban air pollutants increased the permeability of the airways, allowing allergens or histamines easier access to the lung tissues.[16] Another study showed that lungs could be protected from histamine (an inflammatory substance) by an antioxidant nutrient, vitamin C, even when they were exposed to air pollution.[17]

Such chronic free radical effects on the immune system may lead to wide-ranging repercussions. According to Stephen Levine, even low-level exposure, if chronic, may produce cumulative effects on the components of the immune system. When free radicals initiate damage to cell membranes, inflammatory substances such as prostaglandins are released. This in turn can lead to immunosuppression, food and chemical sensitivities, lowered resistance to infection, and eventually degenerative inflammatory diseases, autoimmune diseases, and cancer.

Levine proposes that the free radical theory thus explains how overexposure to environmental chemicals could lead to *ecological illness syndrome,* with its puzzling variety of symptoms. These include irritation of the eyes, nose, lips, and skin; respiratory problems; gastrointestinal problems; fatigue and difficulty remembering or concentrating; headache, weakness, muscle aches, arthritis; and possibly irregular heartbeat and inflamed veins (phlebitis). Although many symptoms seem to be due to "allergies," often they do not involve the formation of antibodies and so do not fit the traditional definition of allergic reactions. (Interestingly, in some people, the symptoms of hypersensitivity are "masked"—that is, the person is free of many overt symptoms—but the underlying condition still leads to an array of degenerative problems.)

Ecological illness, also known as chemical hypersensitivity, is a multifaceted syndrome that begins with exposure to chemicals on the job, in the home, or anywhere in the environment. Levine explains: "Individuals exposed to these chemicals are susceptible to oxidant stresses which can overwhelm the body's protective, antioxidant mechanisms."[18] This excess of free radicals in turn leads to damaged molecules that must be repaired or removed to restore normal function. "If the damaged cellular molecules are not removed or repaired, they may act as persistent, low-level stimuli for abnormal metabolism, altered protein synthesis, mutations, production of autoimmune antibodies, and chronic inflammation."[19] The person becomes hypersensitive to the original compound and to new compounds as well.

Whether or not hypersensitivity is the pathway to such an array of diseases and conditions, Levine and his fellow author Parris Kidd believe that many conditions that plague modern civilization are due to undiagnosed underlying food and chemical hypersensitivities initiated by free radicals, and that a better understanding of them would also help us understand many disease states.[20]

Blumberg, who has studied nutrition and immunity in older people, explains that the immune system has "on" switches and "off" switches. Free radicals tend to shut down the immune system, but antioxidants turn off the "off" switch—in other words, they stimulate the immune system. He notes:

> This is particularly important when we talk about older people who tend to have impaired immune responses—this is considered an age-related change: as you get older, the immune system gets weaker. It turns out that one of the reasons it becomes weaker—presumably because of more free radical reactions or greater sensitivity to them—[is that] you produce more prostaglandins E2 (one of the substances that shuts down the immune system). Vitamin E, for example, inhibits the production of prostaglandins and so you get an immune stimulation.[21]

In support of this theory, Blumberg points to a Canadian study published in 1992 in which the researchers gave an antioxidant-enriched supplement (basically a lot of vitamin E and beta-carotene) to apparently healthy older adults.[22] Since, as Blumberg says, "infection is a major cause of death among the elderly,"[23] applying the results of this study could have a major impact on our length and quality of life. Blumberg says,

> Those who received the supplements had one half the infectious disease episodes; and in those that did get sick the duration was about half as long. That was an exciting study because it was so well done, and is consistent with other studies that have been done in France. And it is also consistent with my own clinical trials where we have looked at the ability of vitamin E to enhance immune response, which it does very faithfully, but we hadn't looked at disease outcomes the way these other studies had.[24]

NEUROLOGICAL PROBLEMS

There is growing evidence that the cells of the central nervous system are particularly vulnerable to free radical damage. The myelin sheath (the white fatty material that encases some nerve fibers)—like the mitochondria—is rich in polyunsaturated fatty acids, which are particularly attractive to free radicals. After a stroke, in which the brain is deprived of oxygen and then flooded with it, or a spinal cord injury, there is massive death of the nerve cells. This is believed to be the result of the free radicals that such trauma provokes.

Oxidation may also be involved in Parkinson's disease, a neurological disease that usually begins after age 50 and strikes 1 in 100 people over age 60. The main symptoms are muscle tremor and rigidity, slow movement, and loss of control over posture. Deterioration progresses for an average of ten years, at which time death usually occurs from infection. A small preliminary study by Stanley Fahn, a neurologist at Columbia University, showed that antioxidant nutrients in large doses may slow the progression of this disease.[25] This finding supports the theory that Parkinson's is due at least in part to the loss of nerve cells from free radical damage, as well as provides the hope that current drug therapy (with levodopa, which has side effects) cannot.

As further evidence that free radicals destroy nerve cells, Stephen Levine argues that people with Down's syndrome and those with Alzheimer's have something in common: premature aging.[26] In the brain neurons of those with Down's syndrome, there is evidence of degenerative changes. This is known to be due to cross-linking of molecules from oxidation, suggesting that accelerated mental degeneration may originate with free radical damage. "This progressive dementia resembles that of Alzheimer's disease," according to Levine. (There is also an association between Down's syndrome and other signs of accelerated aging such as immune dysfunction and higher risk of cataracts.)

In 1992, researchers at the Salk Institute reported preliminary results of an experiment in which vitamin E prevented the death of certain nerve cells. Based on this study and additional experiments using other antioxidant agents, the lead researcher, Dr. David Schubert, concluded "a good diet high in fruit, grains, and vegetables supplemented with extra vitamins E and C as well as beta-carotene—all of which provide antioxidants—may postpone some age-related damage to the brain."[27]

Several other findings support the theory that free radicals affect mental functioning. The brain contains levels of vitamin C that are 50 times higher than in the rest of the body, possibly indicating a strong need for antioxidant protection. When researcher J. M. Carney gave large amounts of antioxidants to aged gerbils, they experienced an increase in neurotransmitters (the chemical messengers of the brain), and a heightened ability to learn.[28]

CATARACTS AND MACULAR DEGENERATION

Age-related ("senile") cataracts and macular degeneration are the major causes of failing vision and blindness as we get older. Cataracts in particular have been well studied and are well understood; they serve as a good model of the aging process because we can measure them accurately, unlike many other aspects of aging.

The lens of the eye is normally clear so that light passes through it. With cataracts, the lens gradually becomes cloudy, distorting and blocking vision. Cataracts are the leading cause of preventable blindness in the world. Each year over seven hundred thousand of them are surgically removed in the United States, making these operations the largest single item in the Medicare budget. Between the ages of 75 and 85, 45 percent of us will be affected by this condition; in the mid-1980s the U.S. Department of Health and Human Services estimated that if cataracts could be delayed by only ten years, the need for cataract surgery would be cut in half.

According to Allen Taylor, who has studied the relationship of nutrients and cataract formation, there is ample evidence that much of the damage to the lens that causes it to become opaque involves oxidation due to exposure to ultraviolet rays, smoking, and normal metabolic processes.[29] Smoking, which appears to create free radical damage, has been associated with cataracts forming in younger people. Ionizing and microwave radiation have also been implicated. And there's no shortage of evidence that antioxidant nutrients—especially vitamin C—reduce the incidence of cataracts, providing additional evidence that cataracts are related to free radical damage.

Macular degeneration is characterized by a slow atrophy of the central portion of the retina. This portion, called the macula, is responsible for the detailed vision we need to read, thread a needle, or recognize people's faces, and for depth perception. As is the case with cataracts, there is substantial evidence that macular degeneration involves excessive exposure to light and free radicals, particularly those found in cigarette smoke. Lipofuscin—the residue of fats and proteins damaged by oxidation—accumulates in and appears to erode certain cells in the macula, beginning a gradual and steady withering of both form and function. Once again, studies showing the protective effect of several antioxidants add credence to the role of free radicals in the degeneration of the aging eye.

ARTHRITIS

Rheumatoid arthritis is a chronic, systemic inflammatory disease in which the synovial membrane that lines and lubricates the joints becomes inflamed and thickened. This erodes the bone underneath, and the joints eventually become swollen, painful, and deformed. The disease also attacks surrounding muscles, tendons, ligaments, and blood vessels. Rheumatoid arthritis has systemic symptoms including weakness, fatigue, fever, and loss of appetite. This form of arthritis is thought to involve autoimmune reactions, and numerous studies have provided evidence that free radical damage occurs to the cells in the joint.

DIABETES

Some researchers believe that certain people have weak antioxidant defenses in cells of the pancreas. As a result, these cells die or lose their ability to produce insulin, thus leading to adult-onset diabetes. In addition, oxidative stress may also be related to the development of complications arising from diabetes. Studies using antioxidants indicate that they offer a new therapeutic approach toward controlling the long-term complications of diabetes.

OSTEOPOROSIS
Research conducted at the University of Texas Health Center in San Antonio suggests that free radicals encourage bones to lose calcium and that superoxide dismutase stops the loss.[30]

A "Unified Disease Theory"?

Is it really possible that so many seemingly unrelated diseases—cancer, heart disease, chemical sensitivities, neurological disease, and arthritis—share the same common denominator: free radical damage? More and more researchers are coming to the conclusion that the accumulating research shows that a toxic buildup of free radicals underlies many diseases and conditions.

As Dr. Hari Sharma sees it, "A decade ago it might have seemed absurd to argue" that such a wide range of diseases could have one basic source of damage.[31] "But now," he believes, "the evidence for this unified understanding is compelling. For most of aging and disease, free radicals form the common link in the causal chain . . . the clinical presentation of different diseases may be due not to different causal mechanisms, but to variations in the protection provided by the body's antioxidant defenses. . . . Under oxidative stress, the weakest link in the body will give way."[32]

Stephen Levine has developed a comprehensive theory of free radical damage and degenerative disease. We've heard the theory that free radicals could be the basis for chemical hypersensitivity. Here's a fuller look at how he explains his unified theory of degenerative disease through the body's ability to "adapt" to free radicals and eventually grow "tolerant."

TOLERANCE AND ADAPTATION

Levine became interested in free radicals and antioxidant biochemistry after he became seriously ill in 1976. Three years later, his problem was finally diagnosed as ecological illness, an increasingly common condition in which the body becomes hypersensitive to a myriad of modern-day chemicals. In his case, this included car exhaust, cigarette smoke, chlorine in tap water, hydrocarbons released from the tar used in road construction, glues, and perfumes. Almost totally incapacitated, Levine was unable to work, and moved to a wooden shack in order to be able to avoid all triggering chemicals for several months.

He began taking selenium-containing kelp supplements because of evidence that they could enhance immunity and reduce inflammation. Some months later, he had recovered, and after much study came to believe that not only are antioxidants useful in treating ecological illness, but that free radical damage could be the basis for understanding a host of other disease processes.

Levine and Parris Kidd, Ph.D., together undertook the immense job of evaluating and integrating hundreds of research and medical findings from a variety of studies of air pollution chemistry, free radical biochemistry, cancer research, and clinical observations relating to cancer and ecological illness among others. In their technical book *Antioxidant Adaptation,* originally published in 1985, as well as in numerous articles, they relate a variety of illnesses to a hypothesis based on free radical damage.[33]

This hypothesis is rooted in the observation that the antioxidant defense system appears to consist of many inter-related, interregulated, and integrated mechanisms that are able to protect tissues from increases in free radical activities. Levine and Kidd learned that exposure to ozone, cigarette smoke, and other inhaled chemicals increases antioxidants in the lungs of laboratory rodents. Such animals are said to have developed a *tolerance* to the oxidant. When they are exposed again to the ozone, they can survive levels that would have been lethal if they had not been exposed previously.

A similar state of adaptation may exist in humans who are chronically exposed to oxidents. A study conducted by Hackney and colleagues in 1975 compared Californians living in the ozone-rich polluted air of the Los Angeles basin with Canadians living in an area that had lower levels of air pollution.[34] When the researchers exposed the Canadians to the ozone, they showed greater reactivity than the Southern Californians. This supports the contention that the Californians became adapted to the smog just as the experimental rodents did.

They also discovered that red blood cells have been used as a model to study the effects of oxidative stress on tissue. There are many examples that establish that levels of the antioxidant enzyme glutathione peroxidase (GP) increase in people with hereditary conditions that increase the oxidative stress on red cells, and that oxidative damage affects the cell's ability to function.

This *adaptation* to oxidant stress obviously has the short-term advantage of immediate survival. But Levine theorizes that if the exposure is sustained, the organism's ability to adapt wil eventually become exhausted. The antioxidants are "borrowed" from other organs that are not in immediate danger of severe stress, or are less essential for survival.

As mentioned earlier, acute oxidant exposure in lung tissues markedly increased the activity of GP, and this appears to be a universal marker for at least the initial stages of adaptation. Since selenium is required for the production of GP, the way this element is distributed in the body offers fascinating clues as to which organs are most likely to be vulnerable when the body is under chronic oxidative stress. Studies show that when selenium intake is low, generally the immune system retains selenium—this element is concentrated in the spleen, lymph nodes, thymus, and adrenal glands. In other portions of the body, such as the red cells of the blood, and in the liver, kidney, muscles, heart, pancreas, and thyroid, selenium levels drop.

As oxidant stresses continue and accumulate, our bodies continue to draw on their reserves, robbing some organs of antioxidant protection and of antioxidant nutrients that have many other functions as well. Cells, tissues, and organs become damaged and our normal metabolic functions begin to break down. According to Levine, at this stage we see the beginning signs of chronic acute illness in the form of inflammatory damage in certain organs. Heredity will probably determine how much resilience we have and which tissues and organs are most susceptible and likely to suffer from disease. Certain individuals may develop chemical sensitivities; nutrients may be absorbed with difficulty, compromising metabolic processes further and contributing to a decline in the immune system and a diminished sense of well-being. Thus, a vicious cycle may begin: the GP enzyme itself becomes vulnerable to oxidation because it has lost its "buddies" that normally support it. As it becomes depleted, it fails to neutralize the metabolites of the numerous toxic chemicals normally metabolized by the liver, lungs, kidneys, skin, testes, and bone marrow. In addition, the body, in an attempt to reduce the quantity of free radicals it produces during normal activities, slows its metabolism.

Studies of people without genetic defects also show that chemical oxidants affect GP activity. For example, in a 1981 study by Griffin and Lane, apparently healthy subjects who worked at an oil refinery were compared with others who worked at schools and hospitals.[35] The first group were considered to have been exposed to free-radical-forming derivatives of hydrocarbons while on the job; the second group was assumed to have been exposed less to these chemicals. When their red blood cells and blood plasma were compared, the exposed group had lower levels of selenium than the unexposed group; the activity of their glutathione peroxidase was also lower. This supports the idea that the initial adaptive phase may cause a local increase in antioxidant defenses, but that this will eventually decrease (in the lung and generally) when defenses have become exhausted. Adaptation "will likely have the long-term consequence of reducing systemic reservoirs of antioxidant factors" (if these factors are not replaced in the diet or as supplements), according to Levine.[36]

Drs. Levine and Kidd propose that this progression can be thought of as occurring in four stages. In the *first stage*, we are still healthy, but increasingly exposed to chemicals via air, water, soil, and food. Our defenses become overtaxed and we enter the *second stage*, which they call adaptation to oxidative stress. We are more susceptible to infection, and develop allergies to chemicals; we have less energy and cope less well with emotional stress. When we reach the *third stage*, we are clearly unwell, with a variety of allergies and sensitivities to foods and environmental chemicals; autoimmune diseases may appear. In the *fourth stage*, the body can't repair the damage fast enough and environmental stresses become more and more difficult to handle. This stage is characterized by exhaustion, and a final breakdown is imminent, which may end with cancer, rapid aging, and serious autoimmune disease . . . and eventually, death.

In conclusion, the authors point out that standard medical procedure for inflammatory conditions, degenerative diseases, and subsequent cardiovascular problems is the use of powerful, high-cost drugs, such as anti-inflammatory drugs, calcium blockers, and cholesterol-lowering drugs. These have their own set of unwanted side effects and although many temporarily reduce the symptoms, they rarely address the underlying causes and so cannot effect a cure.

As evidence mounts that free radicals are involved in many disease processes, so does the evidence that nutritional supplements can increase the power of our antioxidant defense systems to protect us against oxidative damage. The next chapters describe these supplements and present the scientific evidence to support their usefulness.

THREE

The Antioxidant Vitamins

■

Vitamins are chemicals our bodies need to build, maintain, and repair tissues; they act as coenzymes that enable enzymes to catalyze metabolic processes that digest, absorb, and convert food into energy. Compared with macronutrients such as protein, carbohydrate, and fat, we require relatively tiny amounts of these micronutrients.

Each vitamin usually has an array of specific functions, but some in particular function as antioxidants. Many antioxidant vitamins also protect or stimulate the immune system. The vitamins that appear to have the most antioxidant activity are beta-carotene, vitamin C, and vitamin E, although other vitamins such as the B vitamins also appear to be part of our free radical defense system. As this chapter shows, evidence is building that the Recommended Dietary Allowances (RDAs) for vitamins may prevent obvious deficiency diseases such as scurvy and pellagra, but that much higher levels are required to maintain optimum immune function and redox balance.

After vitamins have been absorbed, they become part of our "body pool," and may be used immediately or stored for later use. Water-soluble vitamins such as vitamin C and the B vitamins are used or excreted within a short period of time—hours or a few days—and so must be replaced frequently. Toxicities for water-soluble vitamins are therefore virtually nonexistent. Fat-soluble vitamins such as beta-carotene and vitamins A and E remain in the body longer; they are usually stored in the fat, but may also be kept in some organs, in particular the liver. Any toxicity problems that may occur are more likely therefore to occur with fat-soluble vitamins, although you would still need to take very large doses. The ranges given here include those found safe by the Council for Responsible Nutrition, which bases its conclusions on several thorough expert reviews of the literature.

Beta-carotene (Provitamin A)

Beta-carotene is a member of the family of over four hundred carotenoids—pigments that give orange and yellow fruits and vegetables their color. Beta-carotene, or provitamin A, as it is also called, is a precursor to vitamin A (known as retinol); the body converts as much as it needs into the vitamin. Retinol is usually measured in international units (IU); beta-carotene may occasionally be measured in milligrams (mg); 1 mg is equivalent to 1,666 IU.

Since beta-carotene is converted to vitamin A in the body, it is difficult to separate out the different effects of these two nutrients in epidemiological studies based on food intake. Many of the beneficial effects such as cancer protection and immune enhancement appear to be related to antioxidant properties and immune-boosting activity.

Vitamin A is firmly established as being essential in the formation of healthy epithelial tissue, which is found in the skin, the glands, the mucus membrane, the lining of the hollow organs, and all along the respiratory, gastrointestinal, and genitourinary tracts. It is needed to maintain vision, especially night vision, for regulation of cell development (differentiation), and for healthy reproduction and growth. Vitamin A is also a strong booster of the immune system. A drug derived from vitamin A (Retin-A) has been used to treat acne and reduce wrinkles in photo-aged skin. Other vitamin-A-derived drugs are used to treat serious (cystic) acne and psoriasis. However, these derivatives have serious side effects and should not be confused with the natural form of vitamin A or beta-carotene.

Not all of the beta-carotene we ingest is converted to vitamin A, and beta-carotene has important protective functions of its own. It seems it is carotene—not vitamin A—that provides protection against many forms of cancer, heart disease, stroke, and cataracts. Although vitamin A appears to be a weak antioxidant, beta-carotene far outweighs preformed vitamin A in this department.

ANTIOXIDANT ABILITIES

Beta-carotene has been called "the most efficient quencher of singlet oxygen thus discovered."[1] Singlet oxygen is a reactive oxygen species that is not exactly a free radical, but is still highly reactive. (There is no antioxidant enzyme for this reactive molecule.) Unlike other nutrient antioxidants, such as vitamin E, which is tranformed into a less toxic radical molecule after it has done its job, a beta-carotene molecule is able to survive as is after quenching singlet oxygen. A beta-carotene molecule can take care of one thousand molecules of singlet oxygen. This is due to beta-carotene's structure—it is a large molecule, with a long chain of bonds that enables it to absorb the singlet oxygen's energy and then release it as heat. Beta-carotene also directly scavenges free radicals after they have been produced and thus stops a destructive chain reaction.

An animal study done in 1989 found that beta-carotene decreased the number and severity of gastric ulcers; measurements of the antioxidant enzyme activity led the researchers to conclude that the nutrient scavenged free radicals, thus providing protection and adding to the list of probable free-radical-related conditions.[2]

IMMUNE ENHANCEMENT

Vitamin A's ability to enhance the immune system is illustrated in human and animal studies. It can lower the rate of infections, especially of the respiratory system. High doses of beta-carotene may increase the levels of T cells, important cells of the immune system. It has also been found to be especially useful in preventing noninfectious respiratory diseases, including lung cancer in men who smoke. It may also be protective in people exposed to second-hand smoke as well as to air pollution, since both contain similar oxidants or pro-oxidants such as tar and carbon monoxide. Some researchers report that ozone, a component of urban air pollution, depletes vitamin A; since ozone produces singlet oxygen in the body and beta-carotene quenches it, it is logical that beta-carotene and vitamin A would become depleted.

CANCER PREVENTION

In hundreds of laboratory studies in which cells were exposed to carcinogenic chemicals, viruses, or radiation, beta-carotene and vitamin A were able to prevent cells from transforming into cancer cells. In animal experiments, vitamin A has also prevented tumors in animals exposed to carcinogens and delayed the progression of transplanted tumors.

Many studies of human populations from all over the world—in the United States, England, Finland, Japan, Norway, and Poland—show a correlation between diets high in beta-carotene or vitamin A and a lower incidence of many forms of cancer besides lung cancer. These include cancers of the bronchus, endometrium, bladder, breast, prostate, cervix, colon, rectum, and stomach, as well as melanoma (a deadly form of skin cancer). The results vary from an eightfold decrease in lung cancer to an 80 percent decrease in cancer of the cervix.

In 1991, Regina Ziegler reviewed human studies that looked at beta-carotene and cancer risk. She found that "low intake of vegetables, fruits, and carotenoids is consistently associated with increased lung cancer," as are low levels of beta-carotene in blood serum and plasma.[3] Lung cancer, states Ziegler, has been studied most intensively because it is so prevalent and because epidemiological studies indicate that diet may be involved in its development. She concluded that the evidence strongly suggests an effect for other cancers as well, such as cancers of the mouth, pharynx, larynx, esophagus, stomach, colon, rectum, bladder, and cervix.

According to Zeigler, the earliest prospective study on the relationship between carotenoid intake and cancer was published relatively recently, in 1979. "Previously cancer research had focused on vitamin A and the chemically similar retinoids because of the traditional importance of vitamin A in normal [cell] differentiation and the efficacy of retinoids in limiting carcinogenesis in animal experiments. But β-carotene is itself an antioxidant and has the potential to protect membranes, DNA, and other cellular constituents from oxidative damage."[4]

Other carotenoids also act as antioxidants and may also be involved in preventing cancer. Five to ten different carotenoids have been found in blood serum, with lycopene occurring at the highest concentration. More research is needed, however. According to Ziegler, "What needs to be more carefully examined is the range of carotenoid intake over which an effect is observed." She also suggests that future research examine whether vegetables, fruits, and carotenoids reduce the risk of cancer only in people with nutritionally inadequate diets, or whether increased intake of these substances benefits so-called "well-nourished" individuals as well.

Vitamin A and its derivatives may also affect an already established cancer or precancer. According to work done by Harinder S. Garewal (1992), high-dose vitamin A has been known to reverse leukoplakia, precancerous lesions in the mouth that may lead to cancer.[5] However, at such high doses, there are problems with toxicity; beta-carotene, because of its lack of toxicity, is also being tested either alone or in combination with retinoic acid.

A recent report of a trial using retinoic acid in patients with early- and late-stage head and neck cancer showed a remarkable reduction in the number of second primary (new) tumors; however, it did not show a significant reduction in the recurrence of the original tumor.[6] Animal studies suggest that vitamin A can slow the spread of an existing breast cancer.[7] Researchers at the Arizona Cancer Center recently reported preliminary results of a long-term ongoing trial using Retin-A ointment in women with cervical dysplasia. In women with moderate dysplasia, cells returned to normal in 43 percent of those using the ointment, versus 23 percent of those who did not.[8] While this is a topical treatment, and may reflect retinol's role in cell differentiation more than its antioxidant properties, it is another powerful illustration of the nutrient's anticancer ability, and may offer an alternative treatment for women who don't want to use conventional treatment, which can affect childbearing ability.

Retinol or beta-carotene may also increase the effectiveness of cancer chemotherapy or radiation therapy while decreasing side effects. In a study of women with breast cancer, those who had higher levels of vitamin A in their blood responded twice as well to the therapy as women whose levels were lower.[9] Scottish researchers have reported an improved response to chemotherapy in patients with breast and bowel cancer and melanoma, if they have higher vitamin A levels.[10] In addition, when beta-carotene was given to laboratory animals, their radiation therapy was more effective against cancer.[11] Finnish researchers gave a wide variety of vitamin and mineral supplements, including 15,000 to 40,000 IU of vitamin A and 10,000 to 20,000 IU of beta-carotene, to lung cancer patients along with chemotherapy and radiation. Patients who received vitamin A and beta-carotene lived longer and had fewer side effects from their cancer treatment than those who did not.[12]

The National Cancer Institute is currently overseeing several chemoprevention trials of beta-carotene and/or retinol to determine if they can prevent cancer of the oral cavity, skin, lung, cervix, colon, head, and neck; and of synthetic retinol in breast cancer.

CARDIOVASCULAR DISEASE PREVENTION
There are impressive data from epidemiological, biochemical, and animal studies showing that beta-carotene may protect against atherosclerosis by preventing LDL cholesterol from becoming oxidized. The best human data we have comes from the Nurses' Health Study conducted at Brigham and Women's Hospital, in which 87,000 nurses were asked to fill out food questionnaires. The study

showed that those whose diets were highest in beta-carotene had a 40 percent lower risk of stroke and a 22 percent lower risk of heart attack than those who didn't. (Vitamins C and E also reduced the risk of stroke, but not as much as vitamin A.) Women who ate five or more servings of carrots each week had a 68 percent lower risk of stroke than those who ate carrots only once a month. Randomized trials to determine the benefits of antioxidant supplements are now under way.[13]

Confirming evidence comes from another large study, the Physicians' Health Study, which was initially designed to test the hypothesis that beta-carotene might prevent cancer (this ten-year study involving 20,000 physicians is ongoing).[14] Because of the growing interest in antioxidants and heart disease, the researchers examined the effects of beta-carotene in a subgroup of men who had histories of cardiovascular disease. Preliminary data showed that of the 333 physicians in this group, those who took 50 mg of beta-carotene every other day had half as many heart attacks, strokes, and deaths related to heart disease as those who did not take the supplements. Beta-carotene's effects will continue to be monitored in men who did not have a history of heart disease to see if atherosclerosis can be prevented; the results should be available by 1995. (These two studies also looked at vitamin E, which will be discussed later in this chapter.)

Dr. Ishwarlal Jialal, co-director of the lipid clinic at the University of Texas Southwestern Medical Center, conducted a series of studies on antioxidants and atherosclerosis in 1990 and 1991. They showed that beta-carotene, vitamin E, and vitamin C all inhibited LDL oxidation in test tubes, with beta-carotene reducing the uptake of LDL by macrophages 90 percent.[15]

CATARACT PREVENTION

Beta-carotene may help prevent cataracts, in which oxidative damage is thought to play a part. In 1991 Paul F. Jacques, of Brigham and Women's Hospital, published a study involving a total of 112 subjects: 77 with cataracts, 35 without cataracts. He and his team estimated dietary intake based on a food frequency questionnaire for the one-year period preceding the study, as well as supplement use. They also measured the plasma levels of three antioxidants, including beta-carotene. They found that people with low plasma levels of beta-carotene had five times the risk of developing cataracts compared with those who had high levels of this antioxidant.[16]

Jacques's findings support another study published in 1991, which looked at diet only, and found that the risk of developing several types of cataract decreased with higher vitamin A intake.[17] The authors believe that their results "have important implications for delay or prevention of senile cataract formation." In addition, there is evidence that carotenoids also may protect or delay macular degeneration by protecting cells from oxidative damage caused by light.

HOW MUCH BETA-CAROTENE DO YOU NEED?

There is no RDA for beta-carotene, but health agencies, including the National Cancer Institute, recommend that you eat one to two servings of beta-carotene-rich fruits and vegetables per day, which would contain about 9,000 to 10,000 IU. Most people consume only 2,500 IU per day. The RDA for vitamin A has been established at 5,000 IU per day to prevent severe deficiency diseases such as night blindness.

Many researchers and clinicians suggest that to preserve optimum health, higher doses may be required. For those exposed to cigarette smoke or air pollution, for example, a range of 10,000 to 25,000 IU per day is often recommended, with at least half in the form of beta-carotene.[18] The Council for Responsible Nutrition believes an adequate safety margin to be up to at least 10,000 IU of vitamin A daily;[19] and some clinicians suggest that daily doses of 25,000 up to 50,000 and even 100,000 IU are safe (except for infants, children, and pregnant or lactating women) for specific conditions if taken under professional supervision.[20]

Adverse Effects. There has been some concern about the possibility that excess vitamin A could cause birth defects in humans. This is based on the recognized teratogenic (birth-defect-causing) effects of vitamin-A-like prescription drugs. Several agencies have studied vitamin A use in pregnant women; one found that dosages of up to 10,000 IU per day are safe; another found that "the risk, if any, is not known," but that "women who are at risk for pregnancy should avoid taking supplements containing more than 8,000 IU of vitamin A per day." A third reported that high dosages of retinol (25,000 IU or more) per day are not recommended but further stated that "we cannot impute the cause of birth defects to vitamin A based on present knowledge."[21] (There is no evidence that beta-carotene, even up to 25,000 IU, produces birth defects.)

Adverse effects may occur in those who use over 25,000 IU of vitamin A per day for several months. They include loss of appetite, headache, blurred vision, hair loss, dry, flaky skin, and perhaps liver damge. In most cases, these symptoms reverse themselves a few days after vitamin A intake is reduced. (Interestingly, several researchers have reported that vitamin E may reduce the toxicity of high doses of vitamin A; however, this needs to be studied fur-

Best Food Sources for Beta-carotene[22]

Food	Serving	Beta-carotene (IU)
Carrot juice	1 cup	63,300
Carrots	1/2 cup	19,152
Mango	1 medium	8,061
Cantaloupe	1/2 medium	12,688
Persimmon	1 medium	3,641
Apricots	3 medium	1,109
Watermelon	1 slice	1,764
Pepper, red	1/2 cup	2,850
Pumpkin	1/2 cup	27,016
Collard greens	1 cup	3,491
Spinach, raw	1 cup	4,705
Spinach, cooked	1/2 cup	7,395
Romaine (raw)	1 cup	780
Vegetable juice cocktail	1 cup	2,831
Broccoli	1/2 cup	1,740
Squash, winter	1/2 cup	4,357
Sweet potato	1 small	27,823

Amounts are for fresh or frozen fruits and cooked vegetables, unless otherwise indicated.
Preformed vitamin A is found only in animal sources. It is abundant in beef, veal, and chicken liver (3 ounces of beef liver contains 30,000 IU); fish liver oils; eggs and dairy products.

ther before it can be confirmed.[23] Also, vitamin E intake of more than 600 IU daily may interfere with beta-carotene absorption.

Beta-carotene does not cause any of these adverse effects, and that is why many clinicians recommend that most, if not all, of your vitamin intake be in the form of this nutrient. Since the body forms only as much vitamin A as it requires, there is no danger of overdosing. Since beta-carotene is an orange pigment, the only adverse effect is *carotenemia*, a harmless condition that turns the skin slightly orange. This, too, reverses itself once the carotene intake is reduced. Carotenemia may occur in some people who ingest 25,000 IU of beta-carotene; others will see no effect with much higher doses, according to nutritionist Shari Lieberman, Ph.D. Lieberman writes that "pigments such as carotenes are often given to sun-sensitive individuals since the tinting of the skin affords some additional protection against sunburn."[24] Beta-carotene doses of up to 300,000 IU per day for two or more years have been taken by patients suffering from photosensitivity with no evidence of adverse effects.

Vitamin C (Ascorbic Acid)

Vitamin C is also known as ascorbic acid, which means "without scurvy," the classic deficiency disease of this nutrient. But the more we study vitamin C, the more respect it gets, as it becomes clearer that it has many more biological functions that are at the foundation of maintaining health and preventing disease. As Stephen Levine says, "The studies being done show that Linus Pauling was right" in assigning great importance to ascorbic acid's role in fighting colds.[25]

Vitamin C is needed to synthesize hormones and neurotransmitters, detoxify harmful chemicals, metabolize cholesterol, promote tissue growth and repair, and form bones, cartilage, and collagen (the "glue" that holds tissues together).

ANTIOXIDANT ACTIVITIES
Ascorbic acid plays several roles in the immune system and, of course, is a major (and perhaps the predominant)

antioxidant. As a result, vitamin C appears to protect against many free-radical-related conditions and diseases including cancer, heart disease, lung disease, aging, arthritis, cataracts, and birth defects.

Vitamin C fulfills many roles in the antioxidant system. Since it is water soluble, this substance is able to "scavenge" free radicals in the watery parts in and between cells before radicals attack the fatty parts of the cell such as the cell membrane. Vitamin C protects us from superoxide and the hydroxyl radical. It thus protects the cell walls from damage, and the DNA from mutation.

Vitamin C works with other antioxidants to block free radical chain reactions. For example, after a vitamin E molecule has quenched a free radical, it becomes a radical itself; it appears that vitamin C recycles the E radical back into vitamin E. In addition, vitamin C improves the bioavailability of selenium, an antioxidant mineral that is required by the superoxide dismutase enzyme.

CANCER PREVENTION AND TREATMENT

Vitamin C's effect on an already established cancer is questionable. In Linus Pauling's pioneering study (with Ewan Cameron) in 1976, 1,000 terminally ill cancer patients who received 10 g of vitamin C supplements per day lived, on average, 4.2 times longer than 1,000 who received no supplements; some supplemented patients lived 20 times longer.[26]

Between 1978 and 1982, Cameron conducted a follow-up study in which he compared 1,532 incurable cancer patients who did not take vitamin C supplements with 294 who did. The study found that the supplemented patients had a median overall survival time that was double that of the unsupplemented patients.[27] No one has been able to duplicate Pauling's or Cameron's results. And even though test tube studies show that ascorbic acid slows or prevents the growth of leukemia cells, the evidence is still weighted more toward the likelihood that vitamin C lowers the risk of developing cancer in the first place.

Vitamin C counteracts the harmful effects of many environmental pollutants and chemicals found in our food and water. For example, vitamin C has been shown to inhibit carcinogenesis due specifically to nitrosamines and nitrosamides. These cancer-causing chemicals are formed from nitrates found in many processed foods and in cigarette smoke; some cosmetics also contain nitrosamines and in many locations, so does public drinking water. In one study, vitamin C inhibited the formation of nitrosamine in food by 93 percent. Through its antioxidant activity, vitamin C blocks various chemical carcinogens including benzopyrene and organochlorine pesticides such as DDT, dieldrin, and lindane.[28]

In mice who were exposed to nitrite, vitamin C provided significant protection against lung cancers. And in a study by J. U. Schlegel mice who were given a carcinogen experienced significantly fewer bladder cancers when vitamin C was added to their drinking water.[29]

In a number of studies, vitamin C was founded to reduce chromosome damage to workers whose jobs exposed them to pollutants including coal tar, styrene, methyl methacrylate, and halogenated ethers.

Most of the evidence for vitamin C's ability to protect against cancer comes from epidemiological studies that infer vitamin intake from food intake (fruits and vegetables). Gladys Block, a professor of public health formerly with the National Cancer Institute, has published several reviews of the studies and finds that the greatest protection from ascorbic acid was for throat, mouth, stomach, pancreatic, cervical, and breast cancer. She concludes,

"The strength and consistence of the results . . . suggests that there may be a real and important effect of ascorbic acid in cancer prevention.[30]

In seven studies of oral cancer, all but one found that vitamin C had significant protective effects. One recent study found that those whose intake of vitamin C fell in the lowest quartile had 1.7 times and 2 times the risk of oral cancer for men and women respectively. Two studies of cancer of the larynx found that low intake of vitamin C at least doubled the risk of this form of cancer. Cancer of the esophagus has been the subject of several studies, and here, too, a low intake of foods containing vitamin C more than doubles the risk of cancer.[31]

Of the seven studies of diet and stomach cancer, all found statistically significant protection that cut the risks approximately in half for people who ate higher amounts of vitamin-C-rich fruits and vegetables. The mechanism is likely to be vitamin C's ability to block the carcinogenic effects of nitrosamines in the stomach. British researchers recently found that four 1-g doses per day of vitamin C could cut in half the changes in cells that usually precede stomach cancer. Cervical cancer studies also show that women with low dietary intake have double or quadruple the risk of severe cervical dysplasia or carcinoma in situ, or invasive cervical cancer. In one study, women whose daily intake was less than 30 mg (half the RDA) had seven times the risk of cervical dysplasia as those who took in more than the RDA. Furthermore, an intake of 90 mg (one and a half times the RDA) or less increased the risk by 2.5 times over that for women whose intake was greater than 90 mg. Seven studies found a correlation between rectal cancer and low intakes of vitamin C, with increased risk varying from 1.5 to 3.3 times that with higher intakes.

A recent major analysis of dietary factors and breast cancer found that saturated fat was associated with breast cancer, but that, in addition, "vitamin C intake had the most consistent and statistically significant inverse association with breast cancer risk." The authors concluded that if all postmenopausal women reduced their saturated fat intake to that of the lower one fifth of the population, "the current rate of breast cancer would be reduced by 10 percent in postmenopausal women in North America," and that if they increased their fruit and vegetable intake to reach an average daily consumption of vitamin C equivalent to that of the highest one fifth of the population, "the risk of breast cancer . . . would be reduced by 16 percent." Making both changes together would reduce the incidence by approximately 24 percent.[32]

When Block reviewed the epidemiological studies of diet and lung cancer, she found that most had focused on vitamin A and carotenoids. However, there were five that recently examined vitamin C's role that found a statistically significant protective effect.[33] One, conducted in the New Orleans area, included 1,200 people who had lung cancer and 1,200 who did not. Those who consumed less than 90 mg of ascorbic acid daily had one and a half times the risk of lung cancer as those whose diets contained 140 mg or more. Another study, conducted in Hong Kong, found that low intake of vitamin C raised lung cancer risk 2.4 times. In a Dutch study, those who ingested less than 50 mg per day more than quadrupled their lung cancer risk, as compared with those who took in greater amounts. A prospective study followed 870 men beginning in 1960. Over a 25-year period, 63 died of lung cancer. When compared with the men who consumed 100 mg or more of vitamin C, those who consumed less than 60 mg had a 2.8-fold increased risk. The protective effect even held for smokers: a 55-year-old man who smoked one pack per day and had a low level of dietary and supplement vitamin C had a 25 percent chance of dying from lung cancer over the 25-year follow-up, but a high level of vitamin C reduced the chance to 7 percent.

However, many other diet studies do not find such impressive or unequivocal results. As mentioned earlier, it is difficult to separate out the effects of vitamin C from other nutrients, and most studies do not look specifically at vitamin C. In conclusion, Block writes, "Of the 11 lung cancer studies that have specifically mentioned a vitamin C score, 5 have found a statistically significant positive effect, 4 have found effects in the positive direction, but not significant; and 2 have reported no effect."[34] One study, conducted in Hawaii, actually found that Caucasian women who took vitamin C supplements had an increased risk—but this is probably because the questionnaire included supplement use only in the three months preceding lung cancer symptoms; Caucasian women generally are the group most likely to use supplements, and individuals may begin taking supplements when they begin to feel ill or notice subtle early symptoms of disease. In this study, vitamin C from foods alone reduced the risk of cancer.

CIGARETTE SMOKE AND AIR POLLUTION PROTECTION
There is both direct and circumstantial evidence that vitamin C protects against cigarette smoke. In test tubes, isolated human cells are protected against oxidative damage from nitrogen dioxide, a component of cigarette smoke. What happens in the body is less clear. Much research shows that chronic cigarette smoking lowers the levels of vitamin C in blood serum and in white blood cells—by up to 40 percent in those who smoke a pack or more per day. Although the level of vitamin C in the lungs declines with exposure to nitrogen dioxide for short peri-

ods, it increases with exposure to cigarette smoke on a chronic basis. A rise in the levels of vitamin C may be a sign that the lung has adapted to the oxidant stress. This may be a similar effect to that seen in mice who have been exposed to ozone, whose vitamin E in the lung increased at the expense of vitamin E stored in the spleen.

In a series of experiments conducted by researchers at the University of North Carolina and the Environmental Protection Agency, the lungs of healthy young volunteers were lavaged (rinsed with saline water) before and after exposure to ozone and nitrogen dioxide. The cells from the lungs in the wash indicated that the levels of both vitamin C and E dropped after exposure. Nitrogen dioxide reacts directly with vitamin C, and this may be why smokers have low levels of vitamin C and need to ingest more of it.[35]

HEART DISEASE PREVENTION
Vitamin C also protects against heart disease. In many ways it helps prevent the buildup of fatty plaques on the artery walls, thus decreasing a major factor in heart disease risk. It reduces the oxidation of LDL, or low-density lipoproteins, which are considered the "bad guys." In the studies on antioxidants and atherosclerosis mentioned in the section on beta-carotene, Dr. Ishwarlal Jialal, co-director of the lipid clinic at the University of Texas Southwestern Medical Center, showed that vitamin C inhibited LDL oxidation in test tubes. This antioxidant reduced the uptake of LDL by macrophages 95 percent—making it as potent as the drug probucol.[36]

In addition, human studies show that doses of 1,000 to 2,000 mg per day reduce the aggregation (clumping) of platelets as well as their adhesion to artery walls. Vitamin C may help repair damaged artery walls, which also lessens the chance of cholesterol deposits building up.

Several human studies correlate higher blood levels of vitamin C with HDLs (high-density lipoproteins). These are considered to be the "good guys" because they scavenge cholesterol and protect against heart disease. In animal and human studies, increased levels of vitamin C are linked with a reduction in serum cholesterol. One study of people who took 1,500 mg of vitamin C per day found a significant drop in cholesterol levels. It appears that vitamin C helps shuttle cholesterol to the liver, where it is converted into bile acids, which are then eliminated by the bowel. Vitamin C also appears to help reduce injury to the heart in people with a condition called ischemia (deprivation of oxygen), by reducing free radical damage.[37]

Research has also found that patients who already had atherosclerosis and were given vitamin C were able to walk farther than others who didn't take vitamin C, and without pain or breathlessness. Surgical patients who received 1,000 mg of vitamin C every day had half as many incidents of deep vein thrombosis (a blood clot that often forms in the leg veins, breaks off, and travels to a major organ such as heart, lungs, or brain).[38]

IMMUNE ENHANCEMENT

Another way that vitamin C protects against cancer and other diseases is by enhancing the immune system. It accomplishes this through several mechanisms. Animal and human studies have shown that vitamin C stimulates production of white blood cells, which take care of bacteria and viruses.[39] Levels of vitamin C in white cells drop when we have colds or other infections. Vitamin C is also depleted during physical and emotional stress. It is used up rapidly by the adrenals to synthesize stress hormones, and is lowered by surgery, illness, wounds, and injuries. People who have been injured or who have had surgery experience 50 to 70 percent faster recovery when they are given 400 to 3,000 mg of vitamin C (8 to 50 times the RDA).[40] Gum tissue heals more rapidly after dental surgery when ascorbic acid is given before and after the surgery.

Vitamin C seems to be required by the thymus gland, an important component of the immune system where T cells are produced. Ascorbic acid also increases the production of other components of the immune system, such as antibodies and interferon, needed to defend against foreign invaders and cancer cells. Vitamin C has been shown to assist the liver in detoxifying harmful chemicals by stimulating metabolic enzymes. In addition, this helpful chemical has been able to inactivate a variety of viruses and bacteria in test tubes.[41]

This impressive array of activities helps explain why vitamin C supplements enhance immunity in some elderly adults, and why some people who take vitamin C supplements experience colds that are milder and of shorter duration than people who don't take vitamin C. In one recent study, healthy college students were exposed to other students who had colds. Of the healthy students who received 2,000 mg of vitamin C per day, six caught colds; of those who received a placebo, seven caught colds. Not that much of a difference, but those in the supplemented group also suffered much less—their symptoms were two times less severe and their coughs were three times less severe.

Vitamin C's ability to prevent free radical chain reactions and dampen inflammatory immune processes may also explain why it may be helpful in controlling allergies and asthma. Most people with asthma have low levels of ascorbic acid, and supplements have been shown to reduce spasms of the airways. In one study, 500 mg taken before exercise prevented spasms; in another 1,000 mg reduced asthmatic reactions to sensitizing substances.[42]

CATARACT PREVENTION

Vitamin C levels are lower in lenses that have formed cataracts than in normal, healthy lenses. Feeding high levels of vitamin C to guinea pigs and rats has been shown to delay or prevent cataracts. Human population studies corroborate the relationship of low levels of ascorbic acid to cataracts. In one study (1991), the risk for a particular type of cataract in people with low levels of vitamin C in the blood plasma was 11 times greater than in persons with high levels, and those in the mid-range had 3 times the risk of developing this type of cataract. The subjects who had low vitamin C intakes had 4 times the risk of those whose diets were high in vitamin C.[43]

A 1991 study by James M. Robertson of the University of Western Ontario in London, Ontario, involved two groups of 175 people each; one group had cataracts and one group did not. The subjects were interviewed and when the results were compared, the cataract patients were only 30 percent as likely to have taken vitamin C and 44 percent as likely to have taken vitamin E as the group without cataracts. The daily doses of vitamin C were usually between 300 and 600 mg. The authors concluded that "the consumption of supplementary vitamins C and E may reduce the risk of senile cataracts by about 50–70 percent."[44]

Another study, by Paul F. Jacques and colleagues at Brigham and Women's Hospital, considered dietary and supplement intake as well as plasma levels of vitamin C and other antioxidants. They found that people with a low vitamin C intake (which for the purposes of this study was twice the RDA) or a moderate intake had an increased risk of cataracts, in comparison with people with high intakes.[45]

BIRTH DEFECTS AND MALE FERTILITY

Vitamin C may reduce a type of male infertility due to sperm cells clumping together. In one study, sperm stopped clumping in men who were given supplements of 1,000 mg of C per day. Over a dozen of the subjects' wives became pregnant shortly afterward.[46] Sperm counts have dropped alarmingly all over the industrialized world, and increasing exposure to environmental toxins is a suspected contributor. Free radicals may damage the DNA in sperm, and vitamin C could help. Researchers have also found that women who had a low intake of vitamin C during pregnancy had three times the risk of delivering a child who would later develop brain cancer.[47]

PARKINSON'S DISEASE PREVENTION

Stanley Fahn, of Columbia University, headed a study in which high doses of vitamin E (3,200 units per day) and C (3,000 mg per day) were given to men and women with early Parkinson's disease. This group of patients was compared with another group followed elsewhere who were not taking antioxidants. It appeared that the antioxidants were able to slow the progression of Parkinson's disease. Fahn's patients did not need to begin taking medication (levodopa) for their disease until 2.5 to 3 years after the control group. At the time the study was published, three of the antioxidant group had not needed to begin levodopa at all, thus extending the duration of treatment-free time.[48]

ARTHRITIS

Vitamin C's antioxidant, anti-inflammatory properties may be useful for people who are at risk of (or already suffer from) arthritis. Vitamin C is rapidly depleted during inflammation and this may exacerbate damage to the tissues.

HOW MUCH VITAMIN C DO YOU NEED?
Vitamin C is manufactured in plants and most animals and used by nearly all organisms in vital processes. Those few that cannot make ascorbic acid, including humans, are exceptions and must get it from food if they are to survive. Humans are missing an enzyme needed by the liver to make vitamin C, due to a mutation that occurred in an ancestor millions of years ago. Even though this condition normally would have caused death, the originally mutated species survived, probably because fresh fruits and vegetables and animals were available to supply ascorbic acid in the diet.

This evolutionary dependence on diet to provide such a crucial nutrient puts us at risk of not getting all we need every day. But how much do we need? Many studies indicate that for optimum protection we need more than the RDA of 60 mg per day.

Anthropologists have calculated that the typical "caveman" diet provided about 400 mg of vitamin C every day. Another technique, which involves studying the other animals that have also lost the crucial C-producing enzyme, calculates that guinea pigs and primates eat the equivalent of 2,000 mg of vitamin C per day. Under stress conditions, this leaps up to 7,000 to 10,000 mg per day.[49] Still another method of determining vitamin C need is described by Shari Lieberman:

> The optimum intake of vitamin C may be the amount that our bodies would synthesize if we had the enzyme necessary to manufacture it. Animals which produce their own vitamin C have high levels of it in their tissues. Dependent on stress

conditions, other mammals synthesize the equivalent of 3,000–19,000 milligrams per day, when calculated for a human weighing 154 pounds. Maximum body pools (when the tissues become saturated) in humans have been estimated at 1,500 mg per day; others have evaluated it to be 5,000 mg per day for a 154-pound person. It is estimated that a daily intake of 200 mg of vitamin C would maintain a body pool of this size in a healthy individual—*totally devoid of stress of any kind.*[50]

Yet, the official RDA to prevent deficiency disease is an absurdly low 60 mg for adult men and women. An intake of 100 mg is recommended for smokers. It is not hard to obtain these amounts from a healthful diet. Surveys show that the median intake for vitamin C in men is 73 mg; for females, it is 66 mg. However, there is also evidence that large portions of the U.S. population do not approach the RDA. Biochemical measures show that approximately 10 to 15 percent of white males and 20 to 30 percent of black males take in only 10 mg of vitamin C per day. The elderly are less likely to consume fresh fruits and vegetables than young or middle-aged people, and thus are at high risk of obtaining inadequate amounts of vitamin C.[51]

It is estimated that 20 to 40 percent of American women get less than 70 mg of vitamin C per day.[52] Even if we all achieved the RDA levels, many clinicians feel that these are far too low for optimal protection. A recent study suggests they are right.

James E. Enstrom, an epidemiologist at the School of Public Health at the University of California at Los Angeles, in 1993 released the results of ten years of research involving nearly 12,000 people ranging in age from 25 to 74. The men who took in an average of 300 milligrams of vitamin C per day through food and supplements had a 42 percent lower death rate from heart disease and other causes for these ten years than those whose intake was low (less than 50 mg). Unfortunately, women in the study did not enjoy similar benefits.[53]

Experts agree that the optimum daily amount of vitamin C varies considerably from person to person, and situation to situation. Shari Lieberman suggests a range of 500 to 5,000 mg, divided over the course of a day, depending on your family and personal medical history and current conditions.[54] You may want to raise your intake temporarily in times of stress, surgery or injury, or during the flu season, the allergy season, or if you are exposed to cigarette smoke or polluted air. Certain other conditions such as high risk for cancer may warrant even higher amounts. Linus Pauling recommended intakes ranging from 450 to 4,500 mg per day for "the improvement of general health" and "for increased resistance to infectious disease," and cited literature indicating that doses several times higher were safe.[55] The Council for Responsible Nutrition cites data supporting the safety of up to 40 grams (40,000 mg) in schizophrenic patients, 2,000 mg in burn patients, and a variety of other high dosages, and says these reports demonstrate an adequate safety margin for at least 1 g per day in adults.[56]

Adverse Effects: Although large doses of vitamin C may cause kidney stones, the data exist only for people with a history of kidney problems. The only proven adverse effects of high levels of vitamin C are intestinal gas and looser stools—harmless and completely reversible. In fact, some practitioners use this effect as a guide in determining the optimum high dose, and then reduce the amount by 1 or 2 g. Vitamin C is employed when the liver detoxifies drugs and other chemicals. Anyone taking prescription

Best Food Sources for Vitamin C[57]

Food	Serving	Vitamin C (mg)
Cantaloupe	$1/2$ medium	195
Grapefruit	1 medium	100
Strawberries	1 cup	84
Kiwi fruit	1 medium	74
Mango	1 medium	57
Orange	1 medium	70
Papaya	1 cup	87
Watermelon	1 slice	46
Broccoli	$1/2$ cup	37
Tomato	1 cup	34
Brussels sprouts	$1/2$ cup	35
Cabbage (raw)	1 cup	33
Cauliflower (raw)	$1/2$ cup	36
Kohlrabi	$1/2$ cup	45
Pepper, green	$1/2$ cup	45
Pepper, red	$1/2$ cup	95
Sweet potato	1 small	31

(Amounts are for fresh or frozen fruits and vegetables, unless otherwise indicated.)

drugs should consult with a physician before taking high doses of vitamin C.

Vitamin E (Tocopherol)

Vitamin E is also known as tocopherol, which literally translates from the Greek as "to carry and bear babies." Although required by some animal species for reproduction, and concentrated in the testes of humans, vitamin E's early reputation as a "sex vitamin" has never been proven in humans. Vitamin E, also long touted as good for the heart, is finally being given the recognition many experts feel it deserves. Now there is convincing evidence that it protects against heart disease, infection, cancer, cataracts, neurological disease, and premature aging—in part because of its antioxidant and immune-enhancing properties.

ANTIOXIDANT ABILITIES

According to Lester Packer, a biochemist at the University of California at Berkeley, "Vitamin E is well accepted as the first line of defense against lipid peroxidation." It has been shown to protect against damage from radicals, such as the peroxy radical and oxidation products, and to reduce the oxidative breakdown of fatty acids such as polyunsaturated fatty acids (PUFAs). In this way, it helps maintain the strength and integrity of cell membranes.[58]

Vitamin E also protects DNA against free radical attack, which if unrepaired could lead to cancerous mutations, cell death, or faulty cell reproduction, which could hinder cell function. In addition, vitamin E protects the tiny lysosomes within the cells; these contain destructive substances that could harm the cell.

Vitamin E may be required in protecting against airborne oxidants. Research in rats has shown that vitamin E protects lungs exposed to ozone or cigarette smoke.[59] In one human study, when the breath of smokers was measured for oxidation by-products, higher levels appeared than in nonsmokers; however, these levels were reduced when smokers received 800 IU of daily vitamin E supplements.[60] Lester Packer feels that "until the sources of pollution are eliminated, research shows vitamin E may help protect the lungs from damage associated with exposure to common air pollutants."

More evidence of vitamin E's usefulness in stopping free radical damage comes from animal and human studies of ischemia and reperfusion. During stroke and heart attack, the blood supply is temporarily cut off (ischemia); when it is restored (reperfusion), the sudden surge in oxygen causes free radicals to form. Studies show that vitamin E is depleted during this process and that treating subjects with vitamin E helps prevent the damage.

IMMUNITY ENHANCEMENT
Jeffrey Blumberg, Associate Director of the Human Nutrition Research Center on Aging at Tufts University, writes that in experimental models, "almost every aspect of the immune system," including resistance to infection, antibody responses, lymphocyte responses, and phagocytic responses, "has been shown to be altered by vitamin E deficiency and enhanced by increases in tocopherol intake."

In test tubes and a myriad of animal experiments including mice, chickens, rabbits, pigs, dogs, and calves, vitamin E affects immunity. (In fact, several researchers suggest raising the daily tocopherol requirement of calves to 125 IU as a cost-effective way to enhance immunity and increase resistance to disease.)[61]

The exact nature of vitamin E's influence is not yet clear. Many—but not all—of its effects on the immune system can be explained by its antioxidant function. White blood cell membranes are particularly rich in polyunsaturated fatty acids, which are vulnerable to oxidation. Immune response depends on an intricate system of communication between cells that have intact membranes. Vitamin E may affect the immune system by sparing the white cells from oxidative damage, and this has been demonstrated in experiments.

Other immune cells, the macrophages, need vitamin E

to maintain healthy membranes and their invader-devouring activity. In one experiment, the vitamin E content of macrophages declined by 40 percent when they were exposed to oxidants. Studies show that the numbers of two types of white cells (the B cells and the T cells) decrease when vitamin E is deficient. Other studies demonstrate that vitamin E may be of benefit by preventing free radicals from generating prostaglandin, a known immune-system suppressor.[62]

Human studies on the effect of vitamin E on immunity are still limited. The few that exist are small and inconclusive. A worthy exception is a 1990 study by Simin Meydani and colleagues from the Human Nutrition Research Center on Aging at Tufts University. This represented the first double-blind placebo-controlled trial on the effect of vitamin E supplementation on the immune response of healthy elderly individuals. The majority of subjects who received 800 IU of vitamin E (400 IU twice a day) showed significant enhancement of their immune response. The study supports earlier epidemiological studies that indicate a lower incidence of infectious disease in elderly subjects with high levels of vitamin E in their plasma. The authors are encouraged by these results because a single nutrient supplement was so effective, which is especially significant because "dietary intervention represents the most practical approach for delaying or reversing the rate of decline of immune function with age."[63]

PREMATURE AGING

Studies indicate that vitamin E prolongs the useful life of our cells, thus extending the useful life span of our organs. Red blood cells of healthy people who received vitamin E supplements aged less than the cells of people who were not given supplements. When human cells were placed in a vitamin-E-enriched growth medium, they divided and lived much longer than cells grown in other cultures.[64]

Another way that vitamin E's antioxidant abilities slow premature aging is by protecting collagen from cross-linking. When collagen forms these irregular bonds, it hampers normal function, constricts blood vessels, and hinders circulation. One reseacher gave mice vitamin E and lengthened their mean life span, but not their maximum life span.[65]

CARDIOVASCULAR DISEASE PREVENTION

For decades, the discoverers of vitamin E and other clinicians have observed that vitamin E was useful in alleviating the symptoms of poor circulation and heart disease.[66] Several studies indicated that vitamin E could be used successfully in treating angina, atherosclerosis, thrombophlebitis, and intermittent claudication (poor blood flow to the legs, causing pain and weakness). The problem was that often the studies on vitamin E and heart disease showed conflicting or inconclusive results. As recently as 1991, when he reviewed studies on antioxidants and disease prevention, Anthony Diplock concluded that "the literature on correlation of vitamin E status of human subjects with incidence of cardiovascular disease and cancer has been quite severely inconsistent." One explanation for such inconsistencies, he felt, was that when studies rely on measuring the level of vitamin in the blood, the analysis is often delayed so long that the vitamin's instability makes such analysis unacceptable.[67]

Dr. Ishwarlal Jialal's previously mentioned 1990–1991 studies on antioxidant nutrients and atherosclerosis provided a more reliable link. His studies showed that vitamin E (and vitamin C and beta-carotene) inhibited LDL oxidation in test tubes, with vitamin E reducing the uptake of

LDL by macrophages 45 percent—making it as potent as the drug probucol. He then fed a group of normal subjects 800 IU of vitamin E daily for three months. They experienced no side effects; their blood levels of vitamin E increased by a factor of 3.5, and samples of their LDL were less prone to oxidation.[68]

Finally, in May 1993, the results of two huge studies were released and hit the scientific community "like a bombshell," according to one researcher. The results of the two studies, which included more than 120,000 men and women, were published in the *New England Journal of Medicine*. Together, they offered strong evidence that taking vitamin E supplements in doses substantially greater than the RDA can help prevent heart disease. In both studies, initially healthy people with the highest daily intakes of vitamin E had a 40 percent lower rate of heart disease than those whose intake of E was the lowest. These beneficial effects were evident even in people whose cholesterol levels did not change. The researchers concluded that since vitamin E is an antioxidant, it might reduce heart disease because it could protect LDL cholesterol from oxidation. Earlier studies have shown that LDL (the "bad" cholesterol) damages arteries after free radical oxidation. The greatest protection against heart disease was found in those who consumed between 100 and 249 IU of vitamin E a day over the course of two years.[69]

The largest of the two studies, the Nurses' Health Study, included 87,000 women, aged 34 to 59. The men's study, the Physicians' Health Study, was conducted by the Harvard School of Public Health and included 40,000 health professionals, aged 40 to 75.

Researchers are still cautious, however, and would prefer double-blind trials, in which half the subjects receive vitamin E and the other half receive a placebo, and neither the subjects nor the researchers know which is which until the trial is over and the code is broken.

Other recent studies also support the theory that higher levels of vitamin E reduce the risk of coronary disease. The results of a study out of the University of Tennessee, Memphis, were presented in 1993 at the Conference on Cardiovascular Disease Epidemiology. The investigator, Stephen Kitchevsky, assessed the intake of vitamins C and E and beta-carotene in over ten thousand men and women aged 45 to 65 from four areas in the United States.[70]

Using ultrasound, Kitchevsky measured the thickness of the walls of the subjects' carotid arteries, which deliver blood to the brain and whose thickness is used to gauge risk of stroke. Vitamin E showed the strongest protective effects especially among people over age 55. The people who consumed the highest levels of vitamin E had the lowest risk for stroke, especially older males who had high levels of LDL cholesterol.[71] The Finns have also used ultrasound: in a year-long study of 200 men with high LDL levels, the growth of fatty deposits in major arteries progressed more slowly in those with the highest levels of vitamin E. These individuals had the lowest risk for stroke, especially older males who had high levels of LDL cholesterol. There was a 78 percent difference in the thickness of the walls of the arteries, according to the researcher, Jukka T. Salonen.[72] In yet another study, people who took vitamin E supplements had fewer molecules of oxidized LDL circulating in their blood than people with lower vitamin E levels.[73]

A study by A. J. Verlangieri, Ph.D., and colleagues at the Atherosclerosis Research Laboratory at the University of Mississippi found that vitamin E reduced the severity of atherosclerosis in primates, and in come cases actually caused regression of the blockages. The researchers concluded that natural vitamin E (as opposed to synthetic) may be effective in lessening the severity and reducing the rate of atherosclerosis.[74]

Another way that vitamin E protects against heart disease is by breaking up dangerous blood clots without hampering the blood's ability to clot when necessary, as during an injury. Finally, there is some evidence that vitamin E can lower overall cholesterol, while elevating the "good" cholesterol, HDL (high-density lipoprotein). In one study, 500 IU of vitamin E was given every day and subjects' HDL levels increased by 14 percent.[75]

Another large study conducted in 1987 included several population groups across Europe. The study was coordinated from Basel, Switzerland, and provided strong evidence that a low vitamin E level is a large risk factor in both heart disease and certain types of cancer. Interestingly, the study also highlights the difficulty of evaluating the results of studies that focus on the effects of a single nutrient. Since nutrients act together, a certain amount of one (in this case, vitamin E) may be sufficient only if all the other antioxidant nutrients are in ample supply; however, this same amount may not provide enough protection if other nutrient levels are low.[76]

CANCER PREVENTION

Vitamin E may protect against cancer in several ways. As we have seen, it is an antioxidant, and protects cells from undergoing cancerous changes. In addition, from animal and test tube experiments, we know that vitamin E, like vitamin C, can block the formation of nitrosamines, which are potent carcinogens. Vitamin E reduced the incidence of cancer of the skin, mouth, colon, and breast in animals who were exposed to carcinogens.

Unfortunately, there is not much data from human

studies on the relationship between vitamin E and cancer. According to Gladys Block, the evidence is not as conclusive as the evidence for vitamin C or beta-carotene because most questionnaires used in population surveys have not included vitamin E.[77]

In studies that do show a link, it appears that below-normal levels of vitamin E raised the risk of cancer in the breast, lung, and esophagus, as well as precancerous conditions of the stomach. A study on breast cancer found risk increased by a factor of 5; several other studies document vitamin E's ability to reduce breast cysts, which may be linked with future breast cancer. In one study women with dysplasia saw improvement with vitamin E supplementation.

A large study was recently (1991) conducted in Finland, including 36,265 people aged 15 to 99 years from various parts of the country. During the follow-up 766 people were diagnosed with cancer. The researchers found a statistically significant difference in the levels of vitamin E in the cancer patients; subjects with the lowest levels of vitamin E had 1.5 times the risk of cancer as those with higher levels. Nonsmoking men with low levels of vitamin E had almost twice the risk of other nonsmoking men. The link was strongest for gastrointestinal cancers. However, there did appear to be an association in women who had low levels of both vitamin E and selenium; these women had three times the risk of hormone-related cancers, such as breast, ovary, and endometrium cancers.[78] In animal studies, vitamin E has been shown to enhance the ability of selenium to inhibit breast cancer. The authors conclude, "Any preventive effect may depend on the causes of the cancer, which varies for different cancer sites . . . there are probably cancers the incidence of which does not depend on vitamin E intake."[79]

In several studies, diets rich in foods containing vitamin E have been linked with a lower incidence of lung cancer. Although many other studies have not found a protective effect, theoretically, vitamin E could exert an influence through its effect on air pollution and cigarette smoke.

Ozone decomposes in the body and forms fatty acid peroxy radicals, which lead to lipid peroxidating chain reactions. Vitamin E focuses on these radicals to break the chain and prevent membrane damage and cell death. In one study, vitamin E supplements were administered to cigarette smokers and during supplementation samples of their white blood cells were analyzed. The researcher found that the level of oxidants the cells produced was significantly lower than without supplementation.[80]

An animal study supports vitamin E's protective effect against lung damage from smoking. Rats were fed a diet deficient in vitamin E and selenium, and were then exposed to cigarette smoke; one third of them died. But a group that received these nutrients had a death rate of only 8 percent.[81]

There has been only one published experiment (conducted in the mid-1970s by Daniel Menzel) that studied the dose response of vitamin E supplements and oxidation stress from ozone. The volunteer subjects ate a normal diet and were given increasingly higher daily supplements. The researchers studied their red blood cells after one week of no supplementation, after one week of supplementation of 100 IU per day, and after two weeks of supplementation of 200 IU per day. Menzel reported that there was a clear protective effect against oxidative stress with both levels of supplementation beyond that provided by the normal diet alone. However, there seemed to be no added advantage to the 200 IU regimen over the 100 IU regimen. Menzel stated in his article: "It is clear that the current recommended daily allowance based on other symptoms of vitamin E deficiency is inadequate for protection against current levels of air pollution found globally in the air over our cities."[82]

NEUROLOGICAL DISORDERS

Studies have shown that vitamin E, probably because of its antioxidant properties, can slow the progress of disorders of the nervous system. By protecting the fatty myelin sheath encasing nerve fibers from oxidation, this nutrient may prove of value for older people with early Parkinson's disease and possibly those with Alzheimer's disease. It is suspected that damage from free radicals in the environment plays a role in initiating these conditions.

In the study by Columbia University's Stanley Fahn mentioned in the section on vitamin C, high levels of both vitamins E (3,200 IU per day) and C (3,000 mg per day) were able to slow the progression of Parkinson's disease.[83] As a follow-up a large, multi-center controlled trial known as DATATOP evaluated the effect of 2,000-IU daily doses of vitamin E plus a drug (deprenyl) used to treat Parkinson's.[84] Although in this study vitamin E failed to slow the progression of the disease, some researchers still feel it might be valuable in its earlier stages. Adrianne Bendich, of Hoffmann-La Roche, is one of them. She comments:

Every person who was taking vitamin E was also taking deprenyl. . . . This drug had such an enormous beneficial effect that it is easy to understand that we might not see the effect of vitamin E separate from and above the deprenyl. It was disappointing, but the hypothesis is still there—that in Parkinson's disease there is free radical damage. We can't say that we know for certain that there was no effect from the E . . . it might take longer to see an effect."[85]

Recent experiments at the Salk Institute suggest that antioxidants, and vitamin E in particular, may stave off or slow the progression of Alzheimer's disease. Dr. David Schubert and colleagues first showed that even low concentrations of a protein that accumulates in the brains of Alzheimer's patients could kill nerve cells. Then they applied vitamin E along with the killer protein and found that most of the nerve cells survived the onslaught. This was the first time scientists were able to demonstrate that vitamin E could prevent such cell death. Additional experiments have shown that other antioxidant agents can also protect cells. Although these results are preliminary and have not yet been tested in animals or humans, Dr. Schubert believes a good diet supplemented with extra vitamins C and E and beta-carotene "may postpone some age-related damage to the brain."[86]

Other beneficial nervous system effects that may or may not be related to oxidation include epilepsy and tardive dyskinesia. Epileptic children generally have low levels of vitamin E, and a study reported that the vitamin may help control seizures in epileptic children.[87] Symptoms of tardive dyskinesia, a side effect of certain tranquilizers, were reduced by 43 percent in people receiving 400 to 1,200 IU of vitamin E.[88]

CATARACT PREVENTION

Both test tube and animal studies suggest that oxidative stress caused by the accumulation of free radicals is involved in the development of cataracts in people as they age, and that vitamin E is protective.[89] A 1991 study by James M. Robertson, of the University of Western Ontario in London, Ontario, examined the relationship of supplements and cataracts in 350 men and women. The results of this study support an earlier epidemiological study by the same researcher that found that levels of vitamins C and E and beta-carotene were lower in people with cataracts.[90] This study involved two groups of 175 people each; one group had cataracts and one group did not. The cataract patients were only 44 percent as likely to have taken vitamin E as the group without cataracts. The daily doses were usually 400 mg. The authors conclude that "the consumption of supplementary vitamins C and E may reduce the risk of senile cataracts by about 50–70 percent."

ARTHRITIS
Beginning in 1983, animal research showed that vitamin supplements could reduce the levels of free radicals associated with arthritis. Subsequent human studies show that vitamin E works better than a placebo in controlling pain due to osteoarthritis; in one study vitamin E reduced the need for pain medication and improved subjects' ability to move around.[91]

HOW MUCH VITAMIN E DO YOU NEED?
According to Lester Packer, "Research on vitamin E requirements for healthy adults has not been conclusive." He points out that requirements may vary more than fivefold. Animal research has demonstrated that a high polyunsaturated fatty acid intake increases the vitamin E requirement, presumably because PUFAs are so susceptible to oxidation.[92]

The RDA for vitamin E was lowered from 30 IU to 15 IU in 1968 in part because of the difficulty in obtaining 30 IU from the diet alone. However, many data suggest that 15 IU or even 30 IU would not be sufficient to counteract free radical activity. The 1993 studies discussed earlier (see Cardiovascular Disease Prevention) showed that 100 IU of vitamin E per day reduced heart disease by 40 percent. A

1990 study used 800 IU per day to boost immune function in the elderly.[93] And a test that measures pentane, a by-product of lipid oxidation found in the breath, indicates that 1,000 IU per day is needed to significantly reduce oxidation.[94]

So, even though some conservative experts still maintain we need more studies to confirm these links to determine dosages and to ensure long-term safety, others feel there is enough evidence to recommend at least a modest supplementation. Obtaining even the RDA from food is difficult, especially since most vitamin-E-rich foods are high in fat. Even though the evidence may not be conclusive, Bonnie Liebman, director of nutrition at the Center for Science in the Public Interest, is not alone when she says, "I wouldn't dissuade an individual from taking that level [100 to 400 IU] of vitamin E." Many scientists themselves admit to taking vitamin E supplements, including the lead investigators for the Harvard heart disease studies and the Alzheimer's study. When *Consumer Reports* polled leading experts in the field, they found that 6 out of 14 took vitamin E supplements.[95]

The Council for Responsible Nutrition concluded that vitamin E is safe in adults in doses of up to "several hundred" IU per day.[96] However, people taking anticoagulant drugs should consult with their doctors before taking vitamin E. For optimum general health, Shari Lieberman recommends 200 to 800 IU per day. She recommends working up to these dosages gradually to minimize the possibility of any adverse effects (see below) and monitoring by a professional if you have high blood pressure, as tocopherol may cause blood pressure to rise temporarily.

Adverse Effects: With very high doses (over 1,200 IU per day) some adverse effects have been reported, including nausea, flatulence, diarrhea, headache, fatigue, and weakness.

Best Food Sources for Vitamin E[97]

Food	Serving Size	Vitamin E (IU)
Avocado	1 small	3
Mango	1 medium	3
Collard greens	1 cup	4.5
Spinach	1/2 cup	3
Tomato	1/2 cup	3
Herring	2 medium pieces	3
Shrimp	3 oz	3
Eggs	2 medium	3
Oil	1 tablespoon	
Canola, corn		4.5
Olive, peanut		3
Safflower		7.5
Sunflower		12
Almonds	1/4 cup	9
Brazil nuts	1/4 cup	4.5
Filberts (hazelnuts)	1/4 cup	12
Peanuts	1/4 cup	6
Sunflower seeds	1/4 cup	27
Wheat germ	1/4 cup	7.5

(Amounts are for fresh or frozen fruits and vegetables, unless otherwise indicated.)

Other Vitamins

Several other vitamins have antioxidant activity, or play support roles in the antioxidant system. In some cases less is known about their antioxidant roles than is known about the standard antioxidant vitamins discussed thus far, but this does not necessarily mean they are less important in protecting health.

These additional vitamins are primarily the B vitamins:

vitamins B_1, B_2, B_3, B_5, B_6, B_{12}, and folic acid. Vitamin B_2 (riboflavin), for example, is involved in the regeneration of the antioxidant enzyme glutathione peroxidase. In the Nurses' Health Study mentioned earlier, researchers analyzed the effect of riboflavin on stroke in women. They found that when they added riboflavin to the total antioxidant score (vitamins C, E, and beta-carotene), the overall reduction increased from 45 to 54 percent. Vitamin B_5 (pantothenic acid) is modified in the body to a form that has antioxidant properties and reduces liver peroxides in laboratory and animal experiments.

A wide range of vitamins appear to protect against cancer, although we don't always know why. For example, women who have been infected with a virus called HPV-16 (human papillomavirus) are at higher risk for cervical cancer. However, in 1992 researchers at the University of Alabama found out that those who had the highest levels of folic acid in their blood were much less prone to develop precancerous lesions on their cervices. They found that smokers who took daily supplements containing 1,000 mcg (micrograms) of folic acid along with vitamin B_{12} were much less likely to have precancerous lesions in their lungs.

Low levels of vitamin D appear to be linked with cancer of the breast, colon, and prostate. Two epidemiologists at the University of California at San Diego and their colleagues have collected evidence that the rates for such cancers correlate with the amount of sun exposure, the amount of vitamin D in the diet, and blood levels of vitamin D.[98] Test tube and animal studies have proven that vitamin D slows the growth of cancer cells.

Bendich says, "There's a difference between direct and indirect activity. We scientists try to examine the effects of a single individual micronutrient, but all the body processes are impaired when you have any deficit. It's wise to make sure we ingest sufficient amounts of the full range of all vitamins, not just the 'antioxidant vitamins.' "

The RDAs for the B vitamins are quite low—generally around 2 mg (allowances for B_{12}, folic acid, and biotin, another B vitamin, are measured in micrograms). They are most plentiful in whole grains and green, leafy vegetables, as well as meats, fish, poultry, eggs, nuts, and beans. Even so, they may be difficult to get from food, since even enriched processed grains are replenished with only a few B vitamins, creating an imbalance.

The Council for Responsible Nutrition found in general that there are no known toxicities for the B vitamins.[99] Anthony Almada, of Rainbow Light Nutritional Systems, advises taking no more than ten times the RDA without professional supervision.[100] In her book, *The Real Vitamin & Mineral Book,* Lieberman's optimum daily allowance for the B vitamins ranges from 50 to 300 mg (or micrograms, for some). She emphasizes that you must never take high doses of a single B vitamin without increasing the amount you take of all the others. "This is not only because the B vitamins all work together," she explains, "but also because they compete in the intestines for absorption by the body. If you take enormous amounts of one, you might decrease the absorption of one or more of the others, creating a vitamin B imbalance.[101] And thus a deficiency."

While the evidence for the effectiveness of the major antioxidant vitamins—beta-carotene, vitamin C, and vitamin E—is the most compelling, we also know that all the vitamins work together as a team and with other nutrients as well. It would be foolish to concentrate only on antioxidant vitamins because good health and disease prevention require optimum amounts of all the known vitamins to support the functioning of all our body's interdependent systems.

FOUR

The Antioxidant Mineral Cofactors

■

Unlike vitamins, minerals (or trace metals) do not generally function by themselves as direct antioxidants. Rather, they are cofactors that attach to the antioxidant enzymes produced in the body and activate them. Anthony Almada, director of research and development at Rainbow Light Nutritional Systems, explains it this way: "These trace metals are like the ignition key in a car—you can have all the components present and in working order and a tank full of gas, but if you don't have the key, the car won't run. Similarly, without the cofactor, the enzyme is worthless."[1]

The minerals known to function in this way are selenium, zinc, manganese, copper, and iron. If a deficiency in one of these minerals exists, it could hamper the effectiveness of our antioxidant system. According to Almada, a number of studies support the idea that loading up on extra amounts of some of these minerals, particularly selenium, and perhaps manganese and copper, will also stimulate the body to produce more protective enzymes, as well as increase their activity.[2] This new information contradicts the long-held belief that once an enzyme has reached a saturation point, extra minerals will not appreciably add to the protective effect.

The five minerals covered in this chapter are needed to maintain the proper composition of the fluids in our body, to form healthy blood and bones, and for proper nerve function. Minerals are stored primarily in the bone and muscle tissue, so it is possible to build up toxicity if you ingest very high doses.

Selenium

For a long time selenium was unrecognized as an essential nutrient—in fact, it was thought to be quite harmful and able to cause cancer. Now we know that it offers protection against cancer and many other diseases, stimulates the immune system, is an anti-inflammatory, and protects the heart, probably because of the key role it plays in the antioxidant system.

ANTIOXIDANT COFACTOR
Selenium is part of the glutathione enzyme system, which many feel is one of the two most important antioxidant enzyme systems (the other being SOD, or superoxide dismutase).

Glutathione exists in high concentrations in every cell, especially the liver. This is where it detoxifies harmful chemicals. Glutathione completes the antioxidant process begun by SOD; by breaking down hydrogen peroxide, it also scavenges lipid peroxides, a function that protects cell membranes and DNA from damage. People who are born without the ability to create glutathione suffer massive oxidative damage to the brain and die young.

Glutathione molecules each contain four selenium molecules, so clearly this mineral must be available in sufficient amounts for the enzyme to do its job well.

IMMUNITY ENHANCEMENT

Selenium intake influences the functioning of the immune system, and many scientists credit its antioxidant effect for this benefit. When large doses of selenium and vitamin E were given together to experimental animals, antibody production increased up to thirty times. In other animal experiments, high doses of selenium increased immune response to vaccines.[3]

Phagocytes, the immune cells that engulf foreign invaders, are sluggish when selenium is deficient and active when selenium is supplemented. Recall that phagocytes release free radicals in their battles against invaders; if this poisonous process is not well contained by antioxidants, it grows out of control, damaging healthy tissue—and the immune cells themselves. Furthermore, the inflammatory substances called prostaglandins are immunosuppressive and thus reduce immune function. Selenium has been known to be an anti-inflammatory (veterinarians have long used it to treat arthritis in animals).

Levine cites numerous reports that selenium "can reduce and sometimes eliminate all four classes of chemical sensitivities (phenols, hydrocarbons, formaldehyde, and chlorine) in a majority of . . . chemically hypersensitive individuals."[4] As mentioned earlier, Levine himself suffered from hypersensitivity and was helped enormously by kelp-based selenium supplements of 400 mcg (micrograms) daily. He notes, "There are many free radical mechanisms, but the breakdown of peroxide in particular appears to be an important one when you are dealing with toxic chemicals." He believes that "this is an enormous issue, now that we live in a chemicalized world."[5]

Levine notes that reactivity to cat hair has also been seen to lessen in response to selenium supplements, but that food allergies do not, suggesting that "there are some basic biochemical difference(s) between food and chemical reactivity."

CANCER PREVENTION

Hundreds of studies indicate a link between low blood levels and intake of selenium and an increased risk of cancer. In an overview of antioxidant nutrients and disease prevention, Anthony Diplock, a British free radical researcher, wrote that "selenium is emerging as a dietary factor that may prove to be of major significance as a prophylactic agent against cancer."[6] He provides three possible mechanisms for selenium's protective effects: it is a cofactor for the antioxidant enzyme glutathione peroxidase; it is required by the liver's oxidase system that metabolizes chemical carcinogens; and it is toxic to rapidly growing cancer cells. Another theory is that selenium aids in DNA repair after oxidative damage has occurred.

There is much evidence that low levels of selenium can increase the incidence and progression of cancer in animals when they are exposed to carcinogens or are transplanted with tumors. The converse was also demonstrated; high selenium intake in excess of the normal dietary intake was protective.[7] In a breed of rats that spontaneously develops breast tumors, 82 percent of the group that did not receive selenium supplements developed cancers, but only 10 percent of the supplemented rats did.[8] Selenium supplements may also inhibit recurrences in animals who develop breast cancer after an existing tumor has been medically treated. And selenium has retarded the growth of human cancer cells in test tubes.[9]

Selenium and cancer have been the subject of epidemiological studies in many countries all over the world. Areas with selenium-rich soil, high intakes of selenium, and higher blood levels of selenium are all associated with lower cancer incidence.[10] The United States possesses a varied "selenium map," with the soil in some areas high and others low in this mineral. Rapid City, South Dakota, which has the highest level of selenium, has the lowest cancer death rate in the country; Ohio, with the lowest selenium level, has a cancer rate almost double South Dakota's.

Studies indicate selenium is protective against a broad spectrum of cancers, especially breast, colon, and lung; ovary, cervix, rectum, bladder, esophagus, pancreas, skin, liver, and prostate cancer are also affected, as is leukemia.[11] The lower incidence of breast cancer in Japan may be partially explained by the high selenium intake from seafoods and marine products.[12] For nearly 25 years, scientists have observed that cancer patients tend to have low levels of selenium; those with lower than average levels seem to suffer more multiple primary tumors, multiple recurrences, metastases (spread to distant parts of the body), and shorter survival times after diagnosis.

CARDIOVASCULAR DISEASE PREVENTION

Selenium's role in antioxidation may be responsible for its association with cardiovascular health, as may its ability to reduce unnecessary blood clotting. As is the case with cancer, studies from all over the world point to a selenium–heart disease connection.

Finland, for example, has one of the world's highest death rates from heart disease, and a study involving 11,000 Finns showed that those with low blood levels of selenium have three times the risk of dying from this condition as those with higher levels.[13] Patients with the greatest amount of atherosclerosis have been found to have the lowest plasma levels of selenium.[14] In a German study, people with heart attacks had significantly lower selenium levels than their healthy counterparts.[15]

The U.S. area known as the "stroke belt," which encompasses part of Georgia and the Carolinas, has the highest stroke rate and a high rate of heart disease—and the soil is very low in selenium. People living in an area in China with low-selenium soil develop a heart disease called Keshan disease. Characterized by heart enlargement and early death, this condition responds to selenium supplements.

HOW MUCH SELENIUM DO YOU NEED?
The RDA for selenium is 70 mcg for men, and 55 mcg for women. The Council for Responsible Nutrition has documented that doses "well above" these RDAs are safe. The optimum amount needed by any individual probably varies according to living conditions that influence oxidative stress. Exposure to environmental toxins may deplete this mineral as the antioxidant enzyme glutathione peroxidase steps up production to deal with free radicals. Oil refinery workers who ingested an average of 217 mcg of selenium per day (about three times the RDA) were nevertheless found to have low levels of selenium in their bodies.[16]

Several studies have found that the activity of glutathione peroxidase increases as the selenium intake is increased: in one study, a tenfold increase in selenium doubled the glutathione activity.[17] However, most experts don't recommend daily doses higher than 400 mcg.

Adverse Effects: A few isolated cases of selenium toxicity at doses of 5 mg (5,000 mcg) per day and 27 mg per day have been documented. Symptoms included fingernail thickening, hair loss, garlic odor, and fatigue.[18]

BEST FOOD SOURCES FOR SELENIUM
Unfortunately, there are no accurate charts that indicate the selenium content in food, because this varies greatly depending on the soil content. In general, foods grown in coastal and glaciated zones tend to be lower in selenium. The richest sources are fish and seafoods, organ meats, and meat in general (if the original animal's diet was high in selenium). Whole grains, vegetables such as broccoli, mushrooms, cabbage, and celery may contribute useful amounts, again depending on the content of the soil in which the crops were grown.

Zinc

More than 20 enzymes in our body require zinc to function adequately. These include enzymes that produce DNA and RNA, and the antioxidant enzyme superoxide dismutase. Without adequate zinc (and copper), SOD would not be able to sop up the superoxide free radical in cell plasma.

This relationship with the antioxidant system explains in part the important roles that zinc plays in maintaining immunity, controlling inflammation, and other functions correlated with free radical damage. Zinc also is needed to maintain the structure and function of cell membranes, which enables them better to withstand the onslaught of free radical attack.

Signs of zinc deficiency include slow healing, impaired senses (taste, smell, eyesight), loss of appetite, susceptibility to infection, and impaired fertility in men.

IMMUNE ENHANCEMENT
Zinc's role is well established in the immune system, where it is needed to maintain adequate levels of white blood cells and the cells' activity, especially antibody re-

sponse. We know that zinc is crucial for proper immune function by studying animals and people with genetic disorders that impair their absorption of zinc. Cattle with this disorder stop growing, are extremely vulnerable to infection, and die prematurely. Zinc supplements remedy the situation. Humans with an inherited zinc absorption problem also get frequent infections and die at a young age, unless they receive zinc supplements. Not surprisingly, zinc deficiency is associated with shrinking immune organs: the spleen, thymus, and lymph nodes.

The elderly are at high risk for zinc deficiency, and this may help explain why their immune function declines over time. Not only are these individuals at risk for infection, but they also tend to suffer symptoms of autoimmune disease. Supporting this connection, a study in which people over 70 years of age were given 220-mg zinc supplements daily showed improvement in their immune systems. The level of infection-fighting T cells went up, as did their antibody response, when compared with the unsupplemented group.[19]

Zinc is depleted during upper respiratory infections that are accompanied by fever. Zinc lozenges allowed to slowly dissolve in the mouth have been shown to speed recovery from colds and sore throats.

Several animal experiments provide compelling evidence that zinc is an anti-inflammatory.[20] It appears to prevent cells from releasing histamine, a chemical that causes inflammation. Other studies in humans point to zinc's ability to ease symptoms of rheumatoid arthritis in certain people.[21]

Healing rates are also affected by zinc levels. Hospital patients who were marginally deficient in zinc were given supplements of 150 mg per day. They healed completely in 46 days, as compared with the nonsupplemented group, who took 80 days to heal.[22] In another study, zinc-supplemented subjects with gastric ulcers healed three times as fast as those who did not receive supplements.[23]

CANCER PREVENTION

Zinc appears to lower cancer risk in several ways: through immune enhancement, by acting as a cofactor for the protective and repair enzymes, and by strengthening cell membranes. People with many types of cancer have low levels of zinc (often along with high levels of copper). Adding zinc to animal diets reduced the risk of cancer when the animals were exposed to carcinogens.[24]

We also have reports, however, that low-zinc diets can slow tumor growth in animals.[25] This may be due to the fact that in certain situations zinc "antagonizes" selenium; and that zinc is needed by cells to divide and grow— both healthy cells *and* cancerous cells. Using zinc in cancer treatment should only be done in consultation with a physician knowledgeable in nutritional therapy.

Zinc protects the liver from the toxic cleaning solvent carbon tetrachloride, generally found in chemical manufacturing and industrial cleaners and solvents. It prevents the absorption of the toxic heavy metals cadmium and lead, to which we are exposed in drinking water, car and bus exhaust, cigarette smoke, and industrial pollution.

VISION, TASTE, SMELL

Zinc is required to maintain important functions of our sense organs, which tend to fail as we age. This mineral is highly concentrated in the eye, among other organs. Growing evidence indicates that zinc helps prevent macular degeneration (deterioration of the part of the retina responsible for seeing details): subjects with this condition who received 100 mg of zinc twice a day lost less of their sight than the unsupplemented group.[26] Zinc also appears to be needed to activate vitamin A and so may play a role in preventing night blindness. Other eye conditions that zinc may influence are cataract formation and optic nerve inflammation.

Studies also indicate that zinc deficiency affects the taste buds, changing our ability to taste; this is often accompanied by an altered sense of smell.[27] These changes may contribute to the loss of appetite so common as we grow older, since older patients who receive supplementation report a heightened ability to taste.

FERTILITY AND SEX DRIVE IN MALES

Zinc is found in high concentrations in the semen, the prostate, and the testes. Mild zinc deficiency causes a low sperm count and motility; moderate to severe deficiency leads to shrinking of the testes. Severe deficiencies may also cause sexual interest to plunge or disappear. Men with chronic kidney failure who also had low levels of zinc in their blood reportedly enjoyed a substantial increase in potency when they received extra zinc; tests showed a rise in testosterone levels as well.[28]

The author of *The Doctors' Vitamin and Mineral Encyclopedia*, Sheldon Saul Hendler, is a physician who for ten years of marriage tried unsuccessfully to impregnate his wife. As he relates in the book, his sperm count was low and his sperm cells sluggish and malformed. A few months after taking 50 mg of zinc per day, his sperm count was up to normal and his wife became pregnant. He surmises that his exposure to cadmium (he smoked cigarettes), a zinc antagonist, had been interfering with zinc absorption and utilization. This provides an alternative for infertile couples, who may consider zinc supplements in the male before undergoing the invasive procedures offered by infertility clinics.

HOW MUCH ZINC DO YOU NEED?

The RDA for zinc is 15 mg for males and 12 mg for females. Although zinc is widely available in food, many people do not get enough from their diets. Like selenium, food content depends on soil content, and large areas of the United States have zinc-deficient soil. Surveys indicate that in general, people obtain only one half the RDA from their food.[29] Compounding the problem, several conditions and diseases interfere with zinc absorption. So do a variety of drugs: alcohol, steroids, oral contraceptives, and diuretics.

Many experts therefore recommend somewhat higher levels than the RDA, from about 20 mg up to 50 mg per day. The Council for Responsible Nutrition has concluded that it is safe to take in doses of zinc that are several times the RDA, but that attention should be paid to the balance of zinc, copper, and iron, because some reports indicate high doses of zinc could affect the balance of these other minerals.[30]

ADVERSE EFFECTS

Excess zinc causes gastrointestinal symptoms: nausea and vomiting. (It is sometimes used to induce vomiting.) This level of toxicity occurs only with high doses of 2,000 mg or more. Doses up to 150 mg (ten times the RDA) for periods of 4–6 months have failed to produce toxicity, although if taken on an empty stomach, they may produce nausea.

There are some concerns about zinc's possible effects on cholesterol. Short term experiments suggest that 150 mg of zinc twice a day decreases the level of HDL ("good") cholesterol and raises the level of LDL ("bad") choles-terol.[31] However, another study, using 50 mg of zinc per day, showed the opposite effect.[32] In nutritionist Shari Lieberman's professional and personal experience, taking substantial doses of zinc has not been a problem. In spite of taking 100 mg of zinc for years, her HDL level has in-creased and her LDL has dropped.[33] "Of course," she writes in *The Real Vitamin & Mineral Book*, "I take a *balance* of other supplements along with zinc, as well as do aerobic exercise three times a week."

BEST FOOD SOURCES

Zinc is found in almost all foods, but animal-derived foods are richest and contain the most absorbable form. These foods include meat, poultry, fish, seafood, liver, and eggs. Soybeans, peanuts, and whole grains are also fairly good sources.

Copper

Copper (along with zinc) is required by the form of super-oxide dismutase that protects against free radical damage in cell cytoplasm. It is also needed by the quencher mole-cule, ceruloplasmin, an important blood antioxidant.

Copper's role in the antioxidant defense system seems to explain this metal's reputation as a folk remedy for ar-thritis. Arthritis is an inflammatory condition, and antioxi-dants reduce and prevent inflammation. In contrast to arthritic individuals who wore placebo bracelets, those who wore copper bracelets suffered a recurrence of symp-toms after the bracelets were removed.[34] Apparently, the copper in the bracelets became dissolved in sweat and then was absorbed through the skin. Lending support to this theory of the benefits of copper is the finding that people with rheumatoid arthritis have higher levels of copper and ceruloplasmin in their blood, as well as more copper in their joint fluid.[35] It was previously assumed copper therefore was a causative factor in the disease; with our current knowledge of free radicals, it is now thought that the high levels of copper indicate the body is attempting to fight the inflammation. Drugs containing copper complexes have been found to counteract many inflammatory conditions such as arthritis, and copper–zinc SOD has been injected directly into the joints and under the skin to treat inflammatory conditions.

Another antioxidant link is provided by reports of emphysema in pigs as a result of copper deficiency; this is probably related to insufficient ceruloplasmin, which is needed to protect the lung from oxidative damage due to chronic exposure to oxidants in air pollution and cigarette smoke.[36]

Copper has a wide variety of functions in addition to its role in the antioxidant defense system. Hemoglobin, the oxygen-bearing protein in red blood cells, requires both iron and copper. Copper is needed in the production of collagen, the neurotransmitter noradrenaline, and skin pigment (melanin); for bone development; and for a number of enzymes needed for energy production. Copper deficiency increased the severity of infections in animal experiments, and so appears to be detrimental to immune function.[37]

Copper deficiency in humans is thought to be rare; it causes anemia, impaired immunity, and bone disease. At highest risk are hospital patients being fed intravenously because the solution is usually copper deficient.

HOW MUCH COPPER DO YOU NEED?
There is no RDA for copper; however, the "estimated safe and adequate daily dietary intake" for adults is 1.5 to 3.0

mg. Early studies indicated that the average daily copper intake ranged from 2 to 5 mg.[38] However, more recent studies show a much lower average intake—1 mg per day.[39] This is perhaps due to differences in measuring technique, or to an increase in the consumption of processed foods. Only one third to one half of the copper ingested is absorbed; an excess of zinc seems to interfere with copper absorption, increasing the copper requirement. For these reasons, many professionals feel copper supplementation is prudent in most cases, in a balanced ratio with zinc. The recommended ratio of zinc to copper is ten to one; since the recommended optimal zinc intake is 20 to 50 mg per day, copper intake should be about 2 to 5 mg. The Council for Responsible Nutrition has concluded that copper supplementation is safe up to 5 to 10 mg per day.[40]

ADVERSE EFFECTS

Overt copper toxicity is rare, but does occur in a hereditary disorder called Wilson's disease. In people without this condition, toxicity may occur when a single large amount is ingested (usually by accident through a hot or cold acidic beverage that has been in contact with metallic copper). The acute symptoms are intestinal irritation, nausea, vomiting, headache, and dizziness. Because the absorptive mechanism becomes saturated, much of the copper remains unabsorbed and is excreted in the bile.

BEST FOOD SOURCES

Foods in which copper is most plentiful include liver, shellfish, meats, nuts, legumes, and whole grains. Copper cooking utensils and water pipes may contribute to the total daily intake for some people.

Manganese

Systemwide manganese deficiencies have not been documented in humans, so most of the information we have about its properties has been gleaned from animal experiments. One theory is that the mineral is so essential that nature has developed ways to prevent a deficiency from occurring. For example, when manganese levels are low, it may be that magnesium is able to take its place in certain metabolic processes, thus saving manganese for metabolic processes where it is irreplaceable.

One of manganese's most important roles is that of cofactor in the form of the antioxidant enzyme superoxide dismutase that is needed by the mitochondria of the cells. Manganese seems also to be needed by the nervous system in the synthesis of dopamine, an important neurotransmitter. Studies have also suggested that manganese deficiency affects immune function: antibody response and activity of several immune cells are stimulated by manganese.[41] Interestingly, every type of tumor that has been examined for SOD has had low levels of the form of this enzyme that requires manganese. This suggests that an absence of sufficient manganese plays a role in cancer and perhaps other degenerative diseases related to free radical damage.

In animals, manganese is known to be required for normal reproduction, glucose tolerance, and healthy bone formation. Manganese levels were found to be abnormally low in women with osteoporosis.

HOW MUCH MANGANESE DO YOU NEED?
There is no official RDA for manganese; however, the "estimated safe and adequate daily dietary intake" is 2 to 5 mg for adults. Even with a manganese-rich diet, it may be dif-

ficult to get optimal amounts from foods, because manganese is poorly absorbed by the body. Many practitioners believe manganese intake should be greater than 2 to 5 mg, and the Council for Responsible Nutrition concludes that up to at least 10 mg per day is safe.

ADVERSE EFFECTS

The occurrence of toxicity for manganese from dietary sources is so rare that is is virtually nonexistent. Manganese toxicity has been reported only in workers exposed to high concentrations of industrial dust, with lung disease and central nervous system problems resulting.

BEST FOOD SOURCES FOR MANGANESE

Foods highest in manganese include nuts, seeds, avocado, seaweed, and whole grains. Fruits and vegetables contain modest amounts, as do milk, shellfish, and organ meats. There is very little manganese in the refined foods that most people eat.

Iron

Iron is found in all our cells, but most of it is found in the hemoglobin of our red blood cells. Hemoglobin carries oxygen from the lungs to our tissues, where it is used for energy production.

Iron functions as cofactor for the antioxidant enzyme catalase. Without iron, catalase can't subdue hydrogen peroxide molecules. However, too much iron can actually encourage free radical production. Unbound iron ("free" iron) that is not sequestered in a protein structure generates the hydroxyl radical. It is theorized that premenopausal women have a lower risk of heart disease than men in their age group because menstruation regularly purges their systems of iron-containing blood. This reduces oxidative damage to cholesterol, which in turn helps prevent atherosclerotic plaques from forming in the arteries.

Iron is also needed by the immune system; iron deficiency is correlated with an increased susceptibility to infection, low white cell counts, and impaired antibody production. But again, too much iron can actually create problems with immunity.

Iron deficiency leads to anemia (too few red blood cells). This condition leads to oxygen deprivation of the tissues, decreases energy production, and thus produces symptoms of fatigue and weakness.

HOW MUCH IRON DO YOU NEED?

The RDA for male adults and women over 50 is 10 mg per day; for females who are still menstruating the RDA is 15 mg per day. Most nutritionists agree this is close to the optimal dosage. Some feel it should be a bit higher: 15 mg for men and 20 mg for women. However, it appears that many people do not obtain even the RDA of iron from their diets. Menstruating women are at highest risk, but it is not uncommon for the elderly, adolescents, athletes, pregnant and lactating women, men, and children to be iron deficient. A study of college students found that only 6 out of 74 were getting the RDA for iron.[42] Premenopausal women have a higher RDA than men (one and a half times), but have a lower caloric requirement, making it quite difficult to supply their needs, even when food is carefully selected.

ADVERSE EFFECTS

Iron has low toxicity; the Council for Responsible Nutrition concludes that iron is safe in doses 3–4 times the RDA.[43] Oral doses of 200 mg (ten times the RDA) may cause nausea, cramping, constipation, and diarrhea in a small percentage of people. The Food and Drug Administration estimates that in most people the lethal dose for iron is 200 to 250 mg per kilogram of body weight (1,000 times the RDA). Most instances of toxic effects are in children who accidentally ingest iron pills. In addition, some people have a genetic condition called hemochromatosis, in which large amounts of iron are deposited in vital organs including the liver, lungs, and heart; this rare metabolic condition puts them at risk for iron overload, which damages the organs.

BEST FOOD SOURCES OF IRON
The best sources are meat (particularly organ meats, such as liver), poultry, and fish; not only are these high in iron, but the form of iron is the most absorbable. Eggs, whole grain enriched breads, leafy vegetables such as spinach, and milk also contain respectable amounts, but only a small percentage is actually absorbed by the body. Vitamin C enhances absorbability from nonanimal sources. An old-fashioned way of getting iron was to pierce an apple with iron nails and let the nails sit in the apple for a day so that the iron was absorbed into the apple flesh. A good amount of iron would be left when the nails were removed and the apple was eaten.

Even though the minerals selenium, zinc, manganese, copper, and iron do not as a rule act as direct antioxidants, they are indispensable components of our antioxidant system. However, we should not lose sight of the fact that these and other minerals also have other important functions. As is the case with the vitamins discussed in the previous chapter, an optimum intake of all the known minerals is needed to protect our health and fight diseases, including those related to free radical damage.

FIVE

Other Antioxidants

■

Besides vitamins and minerals, an enormous number of plant compounds—as well as enzymes, proteins, and other chemical substances—may have antioxidant properties.

Plant Power

Many cultures including the Chinese, Indian, and Native American have a long heritage of using plants and plant materials to treat disease and maintain health. Europeans, too, employ a wide variety of phytochemicals (*phyto* means "plant" in Latin). Herbs and other plant-based remedies are finally catching on in the United States, as their benefits become more adequately demonstrated in studies and clinical experience. According to Robert McCaleb, president and director of the Herb Research Foundation in Boulder, more than five hundred different herbs are sold commercially in the United States. "In many cases," he says, "scientists don't yet understand exactly *how* these herbs work. This is hardly surprising, considering that only recently have they figured out the likely mechanism by which aspirin works."

Many herbs and other plant compounds are known to have or suspected of having antioxidant properties. However, we know much less about them than we do about the micronutrients—the vitamins and minerals—described in earlier chapters. Herbs and other plant foods are a combination of compounds, not single isolated substances. This brings up questions about dosages, efficacy, and safety. Admittedly, much remains to be researched and discovered, but the potential for these substances to affect our ability to reduce free radical damage is great—perhaps greater than with the micronutrients.

The substances described below are those that are the best researched, or have received the most attention in recent years, because their benefits may be due in part to their ability to fight free radical damage.

These substances are available in several forms: as teas (most economical), extracts, tinctures (dissolved in alcohol), powders, and pills. Potencies and product purity can vary considerably, so if you want to use them, it is advised that you work with a knowledgeable health professional and buy your products through a well-established source, be that mail order company, health food store, or your health professional. (Some antioxidants come in more palatable form. Garlic is one, as are various cooking herbs and spices such as rosemary and curry. As we cited earlier, antioxidant compounds called phenols found in grapes and wine may help reduce heart disease.)

Flavonoids (also known as bioflavonoids) are nutritional factors that are not quite vitamins, although they were dubbed vitamin P by Albert Szent-Györgyi, who discovered them. (He also was the discoverer of vitamin C.) There are more than five hundred naturally occurring flavonoids in plant foods, often in the company of vitamin C.

Flavonoids are important, multitalented components of the antioxidant defense system. They are themselves antioxidants that scavenge free radicals directly. They may enhance the absorption of vitamin C and may "spare" its turnover in the tissues. Some studies indicate that vitamin C protects a particular flavonoid called quercetin from oxidation.[1] Some flavonoids bind to metals, preventing them from reacting with oxygen. In human and animal studies, flavonoids have shown anticataract properties.[2]

Flavonoids have a long history as circulation enhancers and capillary protectors. Many studies support these functions and indicate that the compounds strengthen the integrity of these tiny blood vessels and so prevent bleeding disorders such as spider veins, hemorrhages, and frequent black and blue marks. It is theorized that they strengthen the vessels by protecting their cells from oxidation.[3] In addition, by increasing the flexibility of the cell walls of red blood cells, flavonoids assist these cells in squeezing through the tiny capillaries.

In many experiments, bioflavonoids have been shown to squelch free radical formation during the inflammatory process.[4] They are thus useful in the treatment of allergies and asthma, which involve inflammation. Flavonoids appear to fight cancer in animal studies, probably due to their antioxidant properties. Moreover, they also enhance enzymes that inactivate carcinogens, another possible cancer-preventing mechanism.[5] Since they reduce cholesterol and inhibit LDL oxidation, bioflavonoids may slow or prevent atherosclerosis and cardiovascular disease.

Finally, bioflavonoids have been shown to have antiviral and antibacterial activity. In test tubes, animals, and humans they are active against herpes viruses, polio viruses, rhinoviruses (which cause the common cold), and influenza viruses.[6] Cranberries, long touted as a natural remedy and preventer of urinary tract infections (cystitis), in all likelihood owe their reputation to the bioflavonoids they contain.

Nearly all of the plant products described in the following pages contain active flavonoids. Flavonoids are also are found in a wide variety of other plants—fruits, vegetables, and herbs—and in nearly every plant part including the nuts, seeds, leaves, flowers, and bark. Citrus fruits are rich in quercetin and hesperidin; rutin is found in buckwheat. Many bioflavonoids, therefore, are rather easily obtained from the diet—and are perhaps more safely obtained this way than from concentrated supplements. Several flavonoids including quercetin and rutin have been shown to produce mutations in test tube studies of bacteria and mammalian cells, cautions Anthony Almada. How this translates into living animals is still unknown, but supplements should be used very sparingly and cautiously.[7] We do know that quercetin can become oxidized in the absence of vitamin C. Quercetin probably is safe, but we do not yet have as much data on it as we do for the antioxidant vitamins and mineral cofactor supplements, and for now you should avoid the high doses of concentrated supplements.

According to Almada, "There's a lot of exciting scientific material about how powerful quercetin is—it was able to reverse tumor cells back to normal—but the questions with *any* phytochemical are: How well is it absorbed? Does it exert any biological activity? And is it safe?" Almada points out that many of the studies with this flavonoid were either test tube studies or involved injecting it into animals, thus bypassing the digestive system. "In one study, humans were given 4,000 mg by mouth," he continues, "and they detected virtually none of it in the blood.

So the small amount in supplements is not likely to have an effect."

Tannins, a type of flavonoid or antioxidant, are contained in green tea. Green tea is especially rich in tannins called catechins. These may be responsible for green tea's ability to strengthen capillaries, to relieve symptoms of rheumatism, and to protect against radiation damage, cancer, and heart disease. There are over three hundred studies on green and black tea, making this a particularly well-researched plant material. Almada feels that drinking green tea as a beverage is the easiest, most cost-effective way to add antioxidants to your health program; he recommends two to three large cups or mugs a day. Black tea also contains tannins.

Ginkgo biloba is the botanical name for the remarkably long-lived ginkgo tree—its family harks back to the age of dinosaurs and today's trees can still reproduce when they are a thousand years old. The leaves, seeds, and nuts have been used in medicine in several cultures including Chinese and Ayurvedic (Indian). Today, biloba extract is one of the best selling drugs in Europe, where it is used to stimulate blood circulation, particularly to the brain, and to treat age-related disorders such as senile dementia, memory loss, and Alzheimer's. Ginkgo has been shown to improve circulation to the limbs, lower cholesterol, prevent oxygen deprivation to the heart, benefit retinal problems and tinnitus (ringing of the ears), and protect against nerve toxins. The latest research shows it affects neurons directly in addition to improving blood flow.[8] It is a proven antioxidant due to the flavonoid and flavonoidlike substances it contains, and this may explain some of its effects. Ginkgo is one of the better studied plant substances, and has been the subject of more than 400 scientific articles, plus several books and symposia. Robert McCaleb says the concentration and dosage that has proved effective in most studies is a standardized extract of 24 percent ginkgo flavone glycosides, in 40-mg doses three times a day (total of 120 mg).[9]

Astragalus is derived from the roots of a Chinese herb. It stimulates the immune system by increasing the levels and activity of white blood cells. It is used in Asia generally to improve health and disease resistance. U.S. studies show astragalus restores function to cancer patients' damaged immune cells.[10] It also lowers blood pressure, increases endurance, and protects the liver from toxic chemicals. In Japanese studies, eight chemicals made from astragalus have inhibited the formation of lipid peroxides, a type of free radical;[11] astragalus extract is used in Russia to protect against oxygen deprivation and heart attack.

Bilberry is a relative of the American blueberry, and is rich in the flavonoid pigments called anthocyanins. These are known antioxidants; bilberry extract has been shown to limit atherosclerosis, be anticarcinogenic, strengthen capillaries, and improve circulation to the heart and extremities. Bilberry is particularly beneficial for the eyes, and studies suggest it can improve vision and prevent cataracts (when given with vitamin E).[12] Bilberry has been studied for nearly 30 years—mostly in Europe, where it is an approved medicine in several countries. Bilberry extracts produced in Europe are available in the United States and are standardized to contain 36 percent bilberry anthocyanosides; in research studies the dose is usually 160 mg of the extract once or twice a day.

Milk thistle protects against liver damage, radiation damage from X rays, and nerve damage from toxic chemicals. It is available in injectable form in Europe only, where it is a standard emergency room remedy for poisoning of the liver. (Nearly all poisons, including air pollution, chemical fumes, and alcohol, and many drugs, including acetaminophen [Tylenol] affect the liver, the organ that detoxifies them.) Milk thistle's benefits seem to be related to the antioxidant flavonoids it contains.

Milk thistle also appears to stimulate the immune system, and may stimulate superoxide dismutase (SOD) production. Although milk thistle is also available in capsules and tablets, Rob McCaleb prefers a standardized extract of milk thistle seed called silymarin because most of the research uses this form.

Pycnogenol is the name of a patented blend of flavonoids that has been used clinically in Europe for many years and has recently received a lot of attention in the United States. The flavonoids in this substance can be found in a variety of plants: grapes, cranberries, beans, cola nuts, and others. However, the ingredients of the patented product called Pycnogenol are extracted from the bark of the European coastal pine tree. The claims made for Pycnogenol are based on a wide variety of studies and on inferences based on what we know about other flavonoids. Many of these are in a booklet on Pycnogenol, called *The New Superantioxidant-Plus*, by Richard Passwater, Ph.D., a noted biochemist and preventive health care authority.

In countries outside the United States, this product has been commonly used to treat many health problems—to improve circulation, vision, and flexibility; and to slow aging. Other claims include reducing cancer risk, heart disease, and stroke; reducing symptoms of allergies and arthritis; and improving the immune system—all of which have been linked with improving the antioxidant defense system.

In test tube studies, Pycnogenol was 20 times more powerful than vitamin C as a scavenger of free radicals such as superoxides, hydroxyl, and peroxide radicals; and 50 times more effective than vitamin E.[13] In tests of capillary integrity in humans and guinea pigs, Pycnogenol produced a greater and longer correction of capillary leakage than most bioflavonoids. This product's bioflavonoids may play an indirect role in the antioxidant defenses. For example, it is theorized that Pycnogenol contributes to heart disease prevention by protecting vitamin C, which in turn protects vitamin E—both antioxidants linked with prevention of atherosclerosis. In addition, Passwater proposes that by reducing histamine production, Pycnogenol helps artery linings resist attack by mutagens, oxidized LDL cholesterol, and free radicals. Passwater says that researchers usually recommend beginning with a daily dose of 100 to 150 mg of Pycnogenol for 2–4 weeks and then tapering off to 50 mg.

Ginseng has been used in the Orient for more than five thousand years. Because in the past, claims of its powers have been so exaggerated, U.S. scientists have been skeptical; however recent well-designed studies support many of its purported benefits, including that of free radical quenching.[14] Other benefits include lowering LDL cholesterol, reducing atherosclerosis, reducing blood sugar, stimulating the immune system, preventing radiation damage to nerves, improving endurance, and preventing cancer.

Medicinal mushrooms and other fungi are being studied and found to have remarkable health benefits. *Ganoderma* *lucidum* (reishi in Japan) is a mushroom that has been shown to be a powerful free radical scavenger that also lowers blood pressure and cholesterol.[15] While some studies have indicated that *Ganoderma lucidum* is an effective anticarcinogen, others have been inconclusive.

Garlic has antibiotic and antifungal effects. It also protects the heart by lowering the levels of cholesterol and harmful lipoproteins and decreasing the tendency for blood to clot, and has been shown to protect against cancer. Garlic contains many active ingredients, some of which are known or suspected antioxidants; these include vitamin C, selenium, sulfur compounds, and flavonoids. There is one drawback to this phytochemical; as Shari Lieberman in *The Real Vitamin & Mineral Book* warns, "Although fresh raw garlic is the least costly source, it could ultimately prove quite costly in terms of your social life! Many studies used either fresh raw garlic or looked at diets that were rich in garlic and related vegetables such as onions and leeks." She says the deodorized garlic products seem to be as effective, and recommends 200 to 1,200 mg daily (1 to 4 oz of fresh garlic or two to six capsules, depending on their potency).

Other Nutritional Supplements

Coenzyme Q_{10} also known as CoQ, or CoQ$_{10}$, Q$_{10}$, or ubiquinone, is a compound synthesized in our bodies' cells. Like a vitamin, it is a coenzyme essential in the processes used by cells to create energy. It is also a potent fat-soluble antioxidant that scavenges free radicals and strengthens cell membranes. Similar in molecular structure to vitamin E, Q_{10} protects cells and appears to be particularly useful in preventing free radical damage due to ischemia (insufficient oxygen) and congestive heart failure. Q_{10} also appears to benefit people suffering from angina, and protects the heart from oxidative damage caused by Adriamycin, a cancer drug. Other data also indicate that Q_{10} is of benefit in muscle-weakening diseases and in boosting immunity. Doses of 10 to 300 mg have been used in clinical trials, and this amount appears to be safe and effective. Some people have reported gastrointestinal upset, loss of appetite, and nausea when taking doses of Q_{10} in the hundreds of milligrams.

Antioxidant enzyme tablets would seem to be the logical way to get more antioxidant enzymes into the body. Enzymes such as superoxide dismutase and catalase are available in tablet form. However, most researchers feel the enzyme cannot survive the digestive process. Certain foods—such as sprouts (bean, seeds, lentils)—contain SOD, glutathione, and catalase, and some people in the field feel these may be a better source. Others claim that if the pills are enteric coated (coated with a protective substance) this allows the enzyme to pass intact through the stomach acid into the small intestines to be absorbed. "There are a number of huge biochemical obstacles to overcome with ingesting enzymes," according to Anthony Almada. "One is the acid in the stomach; another is absorption across the gut wall," he says. "There are a number of studies that show enzymes can be absorbed intact— this goes against what is generally believed, but would explain food allergies. So enzymes may be absorbed intact, but it's probably in very small amounts."

Amino acid supplements. Not to be confused with enzymes, which are complex groups of proteins, amino acids are the building blocks of protein and can be absorbed from food and supplements. The amino acid L-cysteine is a precursor to the antioxidant enzyme L-glutathione in the body. As an oral supplement, L-cysteine is unstable and can degrade as it is absorbed. However, *N-acetyl-L-cysteine (NAC)* is closely related to L-cysteine, but is more stable and when taken orally may replenish L-cysteine levels in the blood; it may also help get it into the cells and increase cellular glutathione. L-cysteine is an antioxidant in its own right: it inhibits white blood cell superoxide anion production, lowers lipoprotein A, and protects against mercury buildup. It is the antidote of choice for Tylenol overdose, which produces many free radicals in the liver.

Glutathione is a mini-protein composed of three amino acids. It is an important component of the glutathione enzyme system, which includes glutathione peroxidase and glutathione reductase. This system is charged with defending the lung, heart, liver, and blood cells from free radical damage. It also helps improve our immune system, aids amino acid transport, increases oxygen delivery to the brain, detoxifies heavy metals, and aids in the synthesis of proteins and DNA precursors. In Japan, glutathione supplements are used to treat conditions related to free radicals. According to an article in the British medical journal *The Lancet* (December 2, 1989) by Buhl et al, immune-suppressed individuals had 70 percent depletion of this amino acid in their blood, and 40 percent depletion in their lung fluid.[16] Jeffrey Bland writes in *The Nutritional Effects of Free Radical Pathology*: "Increased glutathione levels, along with optimal selenium and riboflavin status, are essential in optimizing the body's free radical antioxidant protection system."[17] Almada points out, however, that "glutathione must be broken down into its components before it can pass through the cell membrane, and then reassembled in the cell. In addition, it is more expensive than NAC, is less well taken up, and is an inefficient source of glutathione."

Taurine is an amino acid that influences mineral metabolism in the cell, which can alter oxidation states. Taurine is a less potent, less efficient antioxidant that quenches hypochlorite, a free radical produced in autoimmune disease and infections.

The evidence supporting the antioxidant effects of the various substances discussed in this chapter is provocative and holds great promise. No doubt support for these somewhat "exotic" antioxidants will continue to accumulate, and we should look forward to hearing about more studies that will help guide us in deciding whether we should add them to our antioxidant program.

SIX

Your Antioxidant Defense Program:

HOW TO FIGHT DISEASE AND MAINTAIN OPTIMUM HEALTH

■

Clearly, if we are concerned about fighting disease, maintaining optimal health, and slowing the signs of aging, we need to pay attention to free radicals and antioxidants. The question is: How can we reduce free radical damage and increase antioxidant defenses in our bodies? What approaches are most effective? What is safe? How should we change our diet? Should we also take supplements? If so, which ones and how much? Should we be concerned about exercise and emotional stress creating excess free radicals?

The growing consensus of the scientific community is that eating a healthful diet, getting the right kind of exercise, and avoiding free radical producers such as cigarettes, tobacco, excess alcohol, drugs, sunlight, and unnecessary x-rays are among the foundations of disease prevention, and that some degree of supplementation in addition is wise. Certainly, managing stress better is advisable for many reasons, including the possibility that stress hormones produce free radicals. These measures are effective and safe, and can improve our health in many ways, including by helping our bodies reduce free radical damage.

Eat an Antioxidant Diet

1. Eat five or more servings of fresh fruits and vegetables every day, emphasizing deep-yellow as well as orange fruits and vegetables, and green leafy vegetables.

Your antioxidant defense program should begin with eating lots of fruits and vegetables because these are good natural sources of antioxidants such as beta-carotene and vitamin C. Epidemiological studies on antioxidants—looking at large populations—have found that, as a group, people who eat foods rich in antioxidants live longer and have lower risk of diseases such as cancer and heart disease.[1] It is difficult to determine from such studies which antioxidant is having a particular effect (and antioxidants act synergistically, further complicating the picture) but the overall effect is clear, and it makes sense to obtain as many of these nutrients as possible in the package that nature provides.

In addition, foods high in antioxidant vitamins and minerals (mainly fruits and vegetables) are also rich in other compounds that may provide additional disease protection. These include fiber (which studies show reduces cancer risk and heart disease), flavonoids (see Chapter 5), and a variety of substances found particularly in cruciferous vegetables (broccoli, cabbage, brussels sprouts) that have been shown to prevent cancer and maintain health. Shari Lieberman points out:

> There are hundreds of thousands of chemicals in fresh fruits and vegetables which are still being discovered and studied

and which—judging by recent discoveries—may work in un-expected ways and be synergistic with the known antioxidants. If we don't know about them, how can we possibly expect to get them from a pill?

Emphasizing food as a nutrient source also reduces the danger of placing too much emphasis on free radical damage as the root of all disease. Jeffrey Bland addresses this issue:

> It's a matter of favor and fashion. When it was thought that cancer was a viral disease, everyone was suddenly a virologist; when it looked like we should know more about the immunological system because of AIDS and everything, everyone became an immunologist. Now everyone looks like they might want to be a free radical physiologist. . . . We need to take a step back—not to get caught up in the microscopic examination of every free radical that is produced in the body but rather look at how free radical production is related to the overall control of the oxidation–reduction reactions within cells, which relates to antioxidants, mitochondrial activity, oxygen utilization, toxin buildup within tissue, and other factors.

2. Limit your intake of fats and fatty foods, and strive for a balance between monosaturated, saturated, and polyunsaturated types of fats.

Keep the overall amounts low (experts vary in their recommendations from 30 percent to 20 percent or even lower), but include some fat in every meal. Anthony Almada says that "if people have a fat-free meal, whole grain bread, nonfat yogurt, and a piece of fruit, and then take vitamin supplements, they will absorb very little of the fat-soluble vitamins such as beta-carotene and vitamin E be-

---

Antioxidant Foods: Color Is the Key

You don't have to memorize the names and nutrient content of all the foods high in antioxidant nutrients—just choose with an eye to color. It turns out that the more color-rich your meals are, the richer they are in antioxidants. So choose a variety of fruits and vegetables, keeping these colorful facts in mind:

Yellow and Oranges	Reds, Purples, and Blues	Greens
Foods: carrots, squash, sweet potatoes, peaches, apricots, cantaloupe, pumpkin, tomatoes, papaya, mango, yellow peppers, oranges and other citrus fruits, curcumin (in mustard and curry)	Foods: red bell peppers, chili peppers, blueberries, red and purple grapes, cranberries, cherries, raspberries, tomatoes, strawberries	spinach, kale, broccoli, beet and turnip greens, kiwi fruit, cabbage, brussels sprouts, green tea, spirulina (sea algae)
Antioxidants: beta-carotene, other carotenoids, vitamin C, flavonoids	Antioxidants: carotenoids, flavonoids, vitamin C	Antioxidants: beta-carotene, other carotenoids, flavonoids, vitamin C

Aim for at least five servings of these colorful fruits and vegetables daily; generally, one serving is one small fruit or vegetable, or one-half cup. Don't ignore your less-colorful fruits and vegetables, such as apples, bananas, potatoes, cauliflower, corn, garlic, and onions. These contain many valuable nutrients—discovered and to-be-discovered—that support antioxidant activity or are otherwise protective.

(Note: This chart was adapted from material supplied by Robert McCaleb, the Herb Research Foundation. Used with permission.)

---

cause the meal has so little fat." Researchers are still discovering the effects of various types of fat in the body, occasionally reversing earlier recommendations. Foods high in saturated fats such as milk and meat were once highly recommended, then polyunsaturated fats were thought to be beneficial in heart disease prevention. Today, many experts recommend that you exclude all hydrogenated fats such as margarine. Almada also recommends using extra virgin olive oil, which contains oleic acids, and fatty fish and seafood, which contain omega-3 fats (trout, oysters, clams, lobster) because they protect LDL from being oxidized, as opposed to corn oil or soy oil, which could actually increase the risk of damage from oxidated LDL particles.

3. Prepare food to preserve nutrients and minimize oxidation.

Fruits and vegetables begin to lose antioxidant nutrients quickly once they have been harvested or cut, or if they are overcooked or cooked in large amounts of water. Lieberman advises that we eat vegetables raw, steamed, baked, or quickly stir-fried to minimize nutrient loss. Avoid deep frying and broiling, which form free radicals in the food. Almada recommends that if you barbecue, you arrange the coals like the two banks of a riverbed, with the food on the rack in between them, so the juices do not drip onto the coals, combust (oxidize), and permeate the meat.

4. Minimize sweets.

Avoid refined sugars, and use honey, maple syrup, or other sweeteners sparingly. Lieberman says, "Many people consume too much fruit, and consequently too much sugar." Almada explains, "Too many foods high in fructose and other sweets can deplete copper from the body, and superoxide dismutase is a copper-dependent enzyme."

Get Regular Exercise

Studies show that exercise increases free radical production and depletes antioxidant nutrients such as vitamin E.

However, there are several reasons that the experts do not suggest we stop exercising. First, exercise is essential for physical and emotional well-being. Second, studies show that intermittent exercisers or "weekend" athletes are the ones who need to be concerned about excess free radical formation.[2]

According to one biochemist, binge exercising may be as harmful as binge sunbathing, and could actually backfire and accelerate the aging process.[3] However, in those who follow a regular exercise program the body learns to adapt to the extra free radicals. It increases the level of antioxidant enzymes produced, and it may also increase conservative mechanisms by which we retain antioxidant nutrients. This adaptation is enough to offset the increased oxidative stress. Several studies, in fact, show that frequent exercisers have a lower incidence of certain types of cancer.[4] Exercising in polluted air, however, may pose problems.

Supplement Your Diet with Nutrients

This is where the views begin to diverge, but even conservative researchers are beginning to change their minds about adhering strictly to the old belief that "you can get everything you need from food."

More and more, the experts are beginning to line up behind progressive nutritionists, who have been arguing for years that in these industrialized, stressful times, the "well-balanced diet" is an unachievable myth. As Lieberman explains in her book, *The Real Vitamin & Mineral Book*, the Recommended Dietary Allowances for the various nutrients set by the United States Food and Nutrition Board are fast becoming outdated as a workable concept.[5] RDAs are not readily obtainable through the diet; they are not designed for the individual; and they only pertain to avoiding overt deficiency diseases, not to maintaining optimal health. What's more, few of us are able to eat a well-balanced diet. Nutrient content of food fluctuates widely, and factors such as stress, pollution, and illness deplete nutrients and increase our need for vitamins and minerals.

If the days of relying exclusively on the RDAs and the diet do seem to be numbered, it is thanks in large part to the two 1993 Harvard studies on vitamin E and heart disease (described in Chapter 3). These studies had such a strong impact for several reasons: they were long-term, followed a large number of men and women, were conducted by a prestigious group of researchers, were published in *The New England Journal of Medicine,* and showed a benefit only if the intake of vitamin E was over ten times the RDA—an amount that was highly unlikely to be obtained from food alone.[6] In the words of William Pryor, "Those two articles fell like a bombshell in the free radical community. I had gotten advance word about the results, but I had no idea they were going to be that strong."[7]

Even so, the editorial accompanying the studies asked: Will vitamin E supplements really work? The author, Dr. Daniel Steinberg, a well-regarded researcher at the University of California at San Diego, felt that although the conclusion was that powerful statistical data suggested that this was the case, we still shouldn't make any recommendations regarding public health policy. The reason is that *no one has done the clinical intervention trials* to determine definitively a dose-response relationship and cause and effect relationship.

Jeffrey Bland says, "This is the nub of the argument (against taking supplements), but my feeling is that this is somewhat of an intellectual flogging of the emperor. I don't think we'll ever have unequivocal proof." He believes that the whole "gold standard" for doing pharmacological intervention trials for drugs is probably not applicable to doing nutritional studies at all. "You can't hold people on controlled diets with nutritional supplements for thirty years, with a placebo group, to find answers to these questions about something that at its worst does no harm."

Although the exact relationship between oxidant damage, nutrients, and certain diseases is still not completely clear, Bland continues: "I think we can say without question that the levels of antioxidants that are present in the standard American diet are not adequate to meet the demands of increasing reactive oxidant species . . . and that RDA levels of specific [antioxidant] nutrients . . . are not adequate to meet the needs of a person who is under those kinds of oxidant stress conditions."

Pryor takes supplements himself and points out that many researchers do too, even though most of them hesitate to recommend that the general public follow suit. "Dan Steinberg doesn't take supplements," he says, "but the Harvard group does." When *Consumer Reports* polled some of the leading experts in the field, they found that 6 out of the 14 they contacted took vitamin E supplements.[8] When a nutrition expert recently asked a roomful of biomedical researchers if they were taking vitamin E, 50 percent of them raised their hands. Perhaps Lester Packer, a prominent biochemist at the University of California at Berkeley, states the case most clearly when he says, "Of course I take them! What do you think? I go to school and then come home and forget what I learned?"[9]

Dr. Pryor compares the steady accumulation of scientific evidence to "the water-drop effect" with the Harvard studies being "a very big drop." He says, "A lot of drops falling will eventually wear a hole in the rock. And the rock in this case is resistance to the notion that vitamin supplementation is a good idea."[10]

Jeffrey Blumberg believes that "a rational nutrient supplementation" can be beneficial. But he cautions:

Nutrient supplements are not nutrient substitutes. They are not a panacea, nor are they a magic bullet. They are one tool that people can use to empower themselves to promote their health and prevent disease. Nutrient supplements are like seat belts, which provide you with some insurance against the risk of injury. They do not give you a license to drive recklessly. Similarly, supplements give you some protection against injury, but they don't say you can eat recklessly.[11]

He says that although there is still uncertainty about how effective these antioxidants are in reducing the risk of chronic disease, "some of the data are very good and I think a decision about supplementation can be made by recognizing some probabilities." For example,

• What's the likelihood of your developing cancer or heart disease? Blumberg says you need to look at family history, your own health history, your life-style: Are you a smoker? Are you a heavy exerciser? Did your father have a heart attack or your mother breast cancer? What is your own individual risk—great, medium, or low?

• What is the chance that this supplement will reduce your risk? For example, the studies out of Harvard and Brigham and Women's show that vitamin E reduces the risk of heart disease by about 40 percent.[12]

These factors together represent the probability of your deriving benefit from antioxidant supplements. Then, advises Blumberg, you have to look at risk—he divides this in two categories:

- Cost. "What if I say you have a probability of benefit of 20 or 30 percent and I tell you that it's going to cost you $25,000 a year? Could you afford that? Then what if I tell you it's going to cost you $25 a year, or $250?"
- Toxicity. "I tell you these antioxidants are innocuous. This factor is zero." Adrianne Bendich agrees about vitamin supplements. Beta-carotene is "safe up to very high doses." Vitamin C is "safe, safe, safe." And vitamin E is "safe, wonderfully safe." She points out, however, that the safety index is much narrower with minerals.[13]

"So," Blumberg concludes, "we're talking about something that is safe, relatively inexpensive, and has some magnitude of benefit depending on your history, life-style and diet, correctness and efficacy of the evidence." The evidence is particularly compelling when you consider the costs of treating an already established condition. Blumberg says,

If you go through the same analytical steps and instead of vitamin C you insert lovastatin [a cholesterol-lowering drug] or a cancer chemotherapeutic drug, you find that the toxicities are high and the costs are extremely high and in many cases the benefit isn't much greater. So when we talk about what this country is concerned about, which is preventive medicine, public health care, and health care costs—I think you end up with a strong suggestion that practicing preventive health in part through nutrient supplementation may turn out to be a powerful tool to use.

1. If you take supplements, begin with a basic, complete multivitamin and mineral supplement.

Nutrients are interdependent and work synergistically, so it's best to insure that you have an adequate supply of all the essentials. Blumberg says, "Taking a multivitamin–mineral supplement formulated at about RDA levels while you are trying to eat more healthfully insures that you are getting an adequate amount." Pryor, who since the 1960s has researched and written extensively about free radicals, says he is trying to take "a responsible and conservative position in a controversial field." He recommends that you start with an RDA-level vitamin and mineral supplement, "by a reputable manufacturer from a place that has a good turnover so you get a fresh supply, and make sure it contains the trace minerals cofactors: selenium, zinc, manganese, and copper."[14]

A related approach is to take a complete supplement containing antioxidants and perhaps other nutrients in amounts higher than the RDA. Almada advises taking a multinutrient supplement, with an antioxidant focus containing substantial amounts of vitamin C, beta-carotene, and vitamin E, and the trace metal cofactors.

Jeffrey Bland thinks "prudence and moderation" are the guidelines, until we learn more. That translates into "somewhere in between the RDAs and heroic pharmacological interventions," and is based upon the vitamin and mineral safety index that is published by the Council for Responsible Nutrition.

Lieberman also generally recommends doses in excess of the RDAs. She argues, "There is ample evidence that for many vitamins and minerals, including antioxidants, amounts far above the RDAs are needed for optimum health." She considers the RDAs to be the nutritional equivalent of the minimum wage. "Yes, they are probably enough to keep you alive," she writes in *The Real Vita-*

min & Mineral Book, "but how good is that quality of life?
And why should you not strive for something better?[15]

2. For extra insurance, add the antioxidant nutrients.
The next level of antioxidant insurance is to take additional amounts of antioxidant nutrients in addition to a
complete nutritional formula. These are available as individual supplements, or as special "antioxidant formulas,"
which usually contain at least vitamin C, vitamin E, and
beta-carotene; some add selenium and possibly zinc; others may contain magnesium and copper, and favonoids or
herbs and such. Pryor advises:

> To make it easy I say take the lowest potency you can buy. For
> vitamin E that's usually 100 IU, for beta-carotene it's 10 or 15
> mg (15,000 or 25,000 IU), and 100 to 500 mg of C. Women or
> men who don't eat dairy products should add 1 g of calcium
> carbonate. So, that's four pills a day, plus calcium, which is
> quite modest.[16]

Others might advocate higher amounts, depending on
your life-style and other risk factors.

*3. Add other antioxidants such as herbs and other plant
materials.*
Although the evidence is not as strong as for the antioxidant vitamins and mineral cofactors, you may want to take
your program to the next level and add more antioxidants.
Anthony Almada recommends green tea as the best single
addition; so does Donald Malins, the researcher who identified free radical damage in the DNA of cancerous breasts.
Pryor's attitude is, "Taking other supplements, including
exotic ones like coenzyme Q, is fine with me . . . some are

pretty expensive, and they may do no good, but they do no harm."[17]

DO SUPPLEMENTS CREATE AN IMBALANCE?

Some biochemists are concerned that taking one type of antioxidant could throw the redox mechanism out of balance and end up doing more harm than good. They have a point: rat studies have shown that loading up with vitamin E causes other antioxidant systems to shut down. In this case, only people who have an inherited inability to detoxify free radicals would benefit from supplements. Researchers are working on developing ways to identify redox-deficient individuals (see Testing, Testing in Chapter 7).

Adrienne Bendich answers: "Theoretically, there is always that potential, but we have not seen any evidence in any of the clinical studies. Nor is there consistent animal data."[18] Jeffrey Bland admits there might be dangers, but only at very high levels of supplementation. He reminds us that radicals are quenched in a series of steps:

> If you have a high level of only one antioxidant, you basicaly use that as a reservoir and you form that as its own free radical, which may not be as harmful as the one you started with, but still has reactivity. Let's say you have a free radical that's been formed by radiation and you've quenched it with vitamin C, which forms an ascorbial radical. But this was not further quenched by a vitamin E, which would ultimately have been quenched by glutathione. Then you might end up with ascorbal radicals, which are in themselves free radicals. Without the ascorbate existing in balance with the other antioxidants to take the molecule the next steps down, you wouldn't end up with a nontoxic molecule.[19]

But wouldn't we still be better off than if the original free radical wasn't quenched at all? Bland answers with another question: "What if the by-products of that secondary radical did other things that damaged other regions of the cell? We're talking shades of gray here. I don't think we know enough in all cases where high levels of antioxidants have been proposed to know all the pluses and minuses." However, he also says:

> The levels that have generally been proposed in the literature that I've seen are not in the range where you would see this happening. But if you're talking about therapeutic levels, like some individuals are using for hepatitis—30 to 40 grams of vitamin C per day—that will have a different physiological effect. What that effect is no one knows. Even 10 grams might have a different effect—but it could be a very powerfully positive effect with some degree of secondary effects for people that are deficient in magnesium, vitamin E, and so on.[20]

Wouldn't this argue strongly against supplementation or in favor of taking all supplements at an equivalently high dose? And what about all the other antioxidants we haven't yet discovered?

Bland says that taking a wide range of supplements "sounds more intuitively logical" than not taking any supplements at all. However, he points out, "That's why a lot of people argue—and I feel rightfully so—for using concentrates of real foods. What's the difference between taking a beta-carotene supplement and eating a pound of carrots? We just don't have the answer right now."[21]

Bland continues, "We're still in the infancy of our learning curve. We do know that the other isomers of carotene, for instance, are more soluble and they may be more lipid-bound and so may be better transported into the cell. Even though they're not better sources of vitamin A, they may be able to increase levels in the cell, and have a greater effect."[22]

In other words: We may not know everything, but why not take advantage of what we *do* know?

If you (in consultation with your health care provider) would like to create your own antioxidant defense program using supplements, the following section will show you how, based on the amount of oxidative stress in your life.

How Much Oxidative Stress in Your Life?

Basic laboratory research does not tell us exactly how much we should be taking of the antioxidant nutrients. So, we must turn to clinical nutritionists to find out what works in their clinical practices. And even here, there is no consensus—the amounts they recommend for optimum health vary greatly from one to another—and this is reflected in the range of doses in the Guide to Optimal Doses on page 147.

However, there is general agreement that certain factors (shown in the Checklist on page 146 and explained in more detail in Chapter 1) raise the oxidative stress from free radicals, creating a greater need for antioxidants if they are to keep apace of the damage.

At this time, there seems to be no single magic bullet— all the antioxidants work synergistically in the body, and you need to take them all together to get the greatest benefit. The main thing that varies for most people is not *what* they take, but *how much* they take: the overall level of supplementation—low, medium, or high—depends on the amount of oxidative stress you are under. Most experts feel that adding exotic antioxidants is too much of a gamble because we know less about them and they tend to be expensive. This is not a risk vs. benefit decision—the risks of supplementation as far as we know are minimal or nonexistent; it is a cost vs. benefits decision—is it worth the money? Someone with AIDS, a diagnosis of cancer, or a strong family history of heart disease should consider taking as many different antioxidants as possible, including the exotic ones. For someone with no personal or family history of killer diseases, the added benefits of going beyond those included in the Guide would not be persuasive in relation to the added cost.

To help you decide where you fall within the range of doses shown in the Guide, first use the Checklist of free radical contributors to assess your degree of risk for redox imbalance. The higher number of risk factors, and the greater their intensity, the higher level of supplementation you'll need. Be sure to consider your entire environment—home, work, and play.

Remember your medical history and current health must also be taken into consideration, as well as your family history. A history of cancer, heart disease, arthritis, and so on puts you at higher risk for future problems. Remember, too, that risk for oxidative damage may rise from time to time—such as when you are ill, or have had surgery, or been injured, or burned or exposed to smoke from fire, or are under any kind of stress. These not only increase oxidative damage, but deplete important nutrients, especially the antioxidant nutrients. Pale skin that freckles and sunburns easily is more prone to photo-aging (wrinkles, sagging, and age spots) and to skin cancer.

Oxidative Risk Checklist

Outdoor air pollution   _____
Indoor air pollution   _____

Alcohol, other drugs   _____
Water pollution   _____
Cigarette smoke   _____
Sunlight   _____
X rays   _____
Airplane travel   _____
Psychological stress   _____
Diet   _____
Exercise level   _____

Tips for Supplement Takers

Here are a few basic guidelines to help you get the most out of your antioxidant supplements.

• Store your supplements in a cool dry place, away from heat and light.

• Since your body can absorb and use limited amounts of a nutrient at any one time, if you are taking higher doses than the RDA it is best to divide the doses over the course of the day. The simplest way to do this is to take approximately equal amounts of everything three times a day, with meals. This insures maximum absorption and utilization, while reducing the chance of indigestion which may occur when supplements are taken on an empty stomach.

• If you are taking supplements in amounts that are several times the RDA, this affords a margin of safety. You have considerable leeway and need not worry that something dramatic will happen if you miss one or two doses, or even a whole day's worth. Even the water-soluble vitamins are stored in the body for about two days. Doubling up the next dose or the next day will probably not do much good, since we can only absorb so much at one time.

Guide to Optimal Doses for the
Major Antioxidant Nutrients

The following ranges reflect a range of views (conservative to progressive) and range of risk levels (low risk to high risk) for free-radical-related disease prevention. If you wish to take higher levels of supplementation because you have an established disease, it is essential to consult a knowledgeable professional.

	Optimum Dosage	Minimum Dosage (RDA)
Vitamin C	500–10,000 mg	60 mg
Vitamin E	400–800 IU	15 IU
Beta-carotene	10,000–50,000 IU	5,000 IU (vitamin A)
Selenium	50–400 mcg	70 mcg
	(50–100 mcg if living in a high-selenium area)	
Zinc	20–50 mg	15 mg
Manganese	15–30 mg	NA
Copper	2–5 mg	NA
Iron	15–20 mg (men)	10 mg
	20–30 mg (women)	
Vitamin B complex	25–250 mg	2 mg or less

• It is unlikely that you will become "dependent" on supplements if you take high doses. If you suddenly stop taking them or drop your dosage, you will not experience withdrawal symptoms, or suddenly develop obvious deficiency diseases. However, it is inadvisable to stop anything "cold turkey" if you have been taking it a long time. Your body will need to adjust to the change, so it is best to taper off gradually. Shari Lieberman recommends "stepping down" the dosage every two weeks until you reach your new desired level of supplementation. As an example, she cites the common practice of increasing vitamin C up to 5,000 milligrams a day during the cold and flu season, and then restoring the dosage to normal by reducing it to 4,000 milligrams for two weeks, and then 3,000 milligrams for the next two weeks, and so on until you reach your goal.

• Travellers needn't worry about temporarily reducing their usual dosage out of convenience; you could safely cut dosages in half for one or two weeks, and then resume the usual amounts when you return home.

• There is some disagreement over whether "natural" vitamins derived from food sources are more powerful than "synthetic" vitamins. Most researchers and clinicians feel that a chemical is a chemical—the molecules are the same so the effectiveness is the same. There is some evidence, however, that some nutrients are more absorbable and active in their natural form (such as vitamin E), or in the company of other naturally-occurring nutrients (such as vitamin C and flavonoids). Bear in mind that many supplements labeled "natural" have some synthetic vitamins mixed in, and that natural supplements and food concentrates are generally more expensive than synthetic nutrients.

• There is also disagreement over the advantages of sustained release formulas over regular formulas. In theory it might be advantageous to have a slow, steady supply of nutrients entering the bloodstream. However, this is not necessarily true in some nutrients, and studies show sustained release supplements may decrease overall absorption. People digest at different rates—one supplement taker was shocked to find several years' worth of undigested vitamin pills when he cleared out his septic tank! On the other hand, some people do find their digestive systems tolerate high doses better when they are in sustained release form, so you may want to experiment.

SEVEN

The Future of Antioxidants

■

If what we know now about antioxidants seems exciting, the future of antioxidants is even more so. This field of research has accomplished much, and seems destined to accomplish much more. Even if it fulfills just a fraction of its potential, we will see significant improvements in our overall health and in the way health care is practiced in this country and all over the globe. We will have at our disposal a potent natural tool for better self-care and disease prevention, and a therapy that complements and improves current modes of medical treatment—and be spending less on health care in the process.

Antioxidants as Preventive Medicine

Some experts in the field are suggesting that antioxidant research may finally provide the fulcrum and the framework for a much-needed "paradigm shift"—a whole new way of thinking about health that is prevention-oriented, rather than treatment-oriented. It could mean that the medical establishment will finally catch up with the American public, seven out of ten of whom are already taking vitamin supplements at least occasionally, according to a recent *Newsweek* poll.[1] In a survey conducted in 1993, one third of Americans had used some form of alternative medical therapy.[2]

In spite of spending more than $900 billion on health care in 1993—the highest expenditure of any country in the world—we do not have the highest life expectancy. Although the number one killer, heart disease, is on the downswing (thanks mostly to changing health habits such as diet), we can still expect 1.5 million heart attacks and 500,000 deaths from them in 1993, according to the American Heart Association. The most recent studies suggest that vitamin E supplementation could cut heart disease risk by 40 percent.[3] Mainstream medicine has failed to stem the tide of cancer, America's number two killer— 526,000 are expected to die of this disease in 1993, and one in three Americans now living will eventually have cancer, predicts the American Cancer Society.[4] According to an article in *Newsweek*, authorities have calculated that if antioxidants are really the basis for the correlations seen in epidemiological studies, improved antioxidant consumption could reduce death in the United States due to cancer alone by one third.[5]

The number of older adults is expected to double to almost 65 million within the next four decades. Jeffrey Blumberg, Ph.D., a researcher from Tufts University and a specialist in nutrition and aging, refers to increasing our "health span" and possibly our life expectancy:

It has been estimated that even a 10-year delay in the onset of diseases common among the elderly would save several billion dollars in health care costs in addition to extending the independence and quality of life of the older person . . . Even if free radical damage is not 100 percent of the story—if it's 50 percent or only 30 percent— if you can account for 30 percent of aging and disease through free radicals *and* if we understand how to combat them with things like dietary antioxidants, I think we have a potentially very powerful tool to come to our aid.[6]

But, of course, this can only happen if the public is informed, and if antioxidant supplements are readily available. Some scientists and government health agencies are still reluctant to endorse antioxidants, and insist we first need more studies to confirm the free radical–disease connection, support the efficacy of antioxidants, and fine-tune the way antioxidants are used. For example, at the conclusion of an antioxidant conference held in London in 1989, Louisiana State University's Dr. William Pryor admitted that there is

difficulty in proving that a given biological effect results from free-radical-mediated processes. Free radicals are so reactive that they cannot be directly observed in biological systems. Thus, we are on the trail of an elusive species, and we must look for its "footprints." . . . There is a need both to validate those that we have and to develop newer methods that are more sensitive and more specific.[7]

We also need to appreciate and better understand the complexity of the antioxidant defense system. At the same conference, Dr. Trevor Slater, a biochemist at Brunel University in England, warned that we need

selective suppression of unwanted free radical reactions rather than a blanket-type total inhibition. . . . Total suppression of free radical reactions in our cells and tissues could lead to harm [since] several important reactions of normal metabolism involve free radical intermediates.[8]

Slater further pointed out that an antioxidant must get to the precise location of the formation of the free radical, not just to the right tissue or even the right cell; it must get there at the right time because the half-life of most free radicals is very short; and it must be in the right concentration so it can compete effectively with nearby cell molecules.

We need to study the known antioxidants as well as seek out additional substances that may be just as important, and perhaps more so. As Dr. Pryor observes, the strongest evidence for an anticarcinogenic antioxidant is for beta-carotene. We still don't understand exactly why; nor do we know much about the antioxidant properties of any of the hundreds of other carotenoids. The National Cancer Institute has approximately two dozen "chemoprevention" trials underway using individual antioxidant nutrients (mostly beta-carotene or retinol derivatives) in doses that are considerably higher than the RDA. Because of the long incubation period for cancer, these are long-term studies—we won't have any answers for 5 to 20 years. There are other "intervention" studies planned or in progress that will attempt to pin down specific nutrient actions, as well as doses.

However, as was mentioned in the previous chapter, Gladys Block, professor, School of Public Health at the University of California at Berkeley, feels that controlled, double-blind prospective nutritional studies are difficult to do, and may not even provide the sort of definitive answers that we rightly demand for drug therapies. Some researchers argue, therefore, that we know enough now to begin to make worthwhile changes in the way we use nutrition that would have an enormous impact on our health and our health care costs. Not surprisingly, one of these is Dr. Block, who said during a 1993 conference on cancer prevention: "Policy makers should back away from the position that you shouldn't take supplements. . . . We must look at nutrition with a new perspective."[9]

Dr. Block found an "enormous gap" between the government dietary recommendations and reality: dietary guidelines generally recommend at least five servings of fruits and vegetables daily; however, a recent survey of 12,000 adults found that only 10 percent had eaten the recommended five servings. Furthermore, 41 percent of the population had not eaten even one fruit on the day of the survey, 17 percent ate no vegetable at all, not even potatoes, and only 25 percent had eaten a fruit or vegetable rich in vitamin C or beta-carotene.

And yet the Food and Drug Administration seems to be biased against supplementation: it wants to limit severely the kinds and quantities of dietary supplements on the market, and has refused to allow a properly qualified health claim on antioxidant supplements informing the public that they may help reduce the risk of some types of cancer. In so doing, the FDA appears to hold antioxidants up to a higher standard than it holds for other health factors such as dietary fats. The 1993 FDA proposed ruling notes that "the effects of different types of fat . . . have not been studied extensively, and the results that do bear on this issue are as yet inconclusive . . . [but] repeated and consistent findings of an association between certain dietary factors and diseases are likely to be real and indicative of a cause-and-effect relationship."[10] Block and many other scientists believe that the evidence in favor of antioxidants' role in cancer prevention is at least as substantial as that in relation to fats, and that it is unfair that the

FDA finds that observational epidemiological studies "are generally accepted as sufficient" for the first Surgeon General's Report on Smoking, and the current proposed ruling on fats, but are not sufficient for antioxidants.

This group of scientists feels strongly that the FDA should reverse its position on antioxidants because of its potential enormous impact on public health. A position paper submitted to the FDA by Dr. Block, co-signed by 11 other scientists and endorsed by another 43 scientists, concludes: "The public good calls for permitting this health claim. If there ever was a case where the error of omission vastly outweighs the error of commission, this is one."[11] And researcher Paul F. Jacques, Ph.D., of Tufts University, asks, "Must we wait for 15 to 20 years to gather sufficient experimental data before taking any action?"[12]

Adrianne Bendich, Clinical Research Scientist at Hoffmann-La Roche, is particularly concerned about the impact that antioxidants could have on the health of the poor and elderly. Her "biggest wish" is that

> when we talk about health care reform we put preventive nutrition very high on the list, and that would include antioxidant supplementation. By that I mean there should be access to supplements from Day One. One of my biggest frustrations is that one out of every ten people in the U.S. is getting food stamps right now. They can use those stamps for potato chips, popcorn, and soda pop, but they cannot use food stamps to buy supplements, including antioxidants.[13]

Bendich points out that "our [government] programs for poor women who are pregnant allow women to get prenatal supplements, but not in between pregnancies. . . . We're twenty-first in the world in infant mortality, and nutrition is one of the major components." She also feels that "elderly people, including those who are in nursing home facilities, should be given information about the importance of vitamins, including the antioxidants, and let them decide if they want to take them. Currently, supplements must be paid for totally out of pocket—not one cent of any co-payments goes toward them."[14]

Antioxidants as Support or Complementary Medicine

Antioxidant therapy may become routine during the treatment of many diseases to slow their progress or help the body heal and reverse the process. Because free radicals seem to be both a cause and an effect, antioxidant therapy may help reduce the free radical damage that is caused by an established condition. In addition, we may be able to counteract the excess free radicals fostered by certain drugs and radiation treatment and so reduce the unwanted side effects.

For example, research shows that antioxidants may be useful for reducing damage from trauma due to stroke, spinal cord injury, and brain injury; reducing damage to the heart muscle after heart attack; lowering the risk of a cancer recurrence in someone who has already had one cancer (evidence for lung, breast, oral, and colorectal cancer); slowing the progress of Parkinson's disease, Alzheimer's disease, and other neurological conditions; protecting the lungs of premature infants; reducing the side effects of many drugs and treatments that form free radicals in the body, including chemotherapy and x-ray therapy for cancer; reducing diabetes complications; reducing the effects of HIV infection; and increasing the success of liver transplants.[15]

Chronic inflammatory diseases are highly likely targets

for antioxidant therapy. Adrianne Bendich discusses the role of free radicals in diseases such as arthritis, Crohn's disease, cystic fibrosis, and acute respiratory disease, which produce free radicals on a chronic basis:

> These free radicals then circulate throughout the body. There is a high degree of oxidative damage in the knees of arthritic patients and studies show that people with arthritis have a lower antioxidant status compared with people who are matched to them for dietary intake. It is the same with a number of other chronic inflammatory diseases. This creates a vicious cycle—free radicals are involved in the initiation of the disease, but then the disease itself creates free radicals and more free radical damage.[16]

Bendich says that free radical researchers such as herself have been talking about what can be done with antioxidants to protect firefighters who are exposed to a very high level of oxidative products on the job—"That's what fires do, they oxidate things." She hastens to admit that "no human studies . . . show this translates into disease." However, she adds, "there are animal models." Animals who have had a part of their bodies burned have high amounts of free radicals circulating in other parts of their bodies, "so this has implications for human burn victims, as well as for firefighters."[17]

Testing, Testing

Another avenue of research seeks to fine-tune and individualize antioxidant therapy so it is less hit-or-miss. Scientists are investigating ways to measure how much damage free radical molecules actually cause and hope to eventually develop tests that measure our antioxidant status and the extent of our redox potential. Stephen Levine asserts that "understanding this oxidation–reduction (redox) state is one way to measure overall health."

In the near future, we may be able to measure free radical damage accurately or measure its by-products as markers for detecting individuals at high risk for developing disease, before it becomes established. Then we may be able to target people who are at especially high risk of oxidative damage—and perhaps treat them with special diets, nutritional supplements, or both. Since individuals vary, tests may also be available that determine how much of any particular antioxidant nutrient is needed by an individual. We may be measuring antioxidant enzyme activity in the blood cells as an indication of oxidative stress, and using this as a tool to evaluate the effect of antioxidant therapy.

William Pryor has defined the term *oxidative stress status*, or *OSS*, and has written several articles on the subject. When he first became interested in developing a way to test for oxidative stress, he was astounded to discover that "there are a ton of ways to measure oxidative status. There were 250 references on the subject." These include testing the exhaled breath, the blood, the urine, the saliva, and body tissues. Pryor is measuring lipid peroxidation by-products, ethane and pentane, in exhaled breath. This method is the least invasive, he says, and "it would be really nifty if it would work because of that." In collaboration with scientists at Johns Hopkins University, Pryor is studying people in a hospital setting, to see if they can predict who should have high oxidative stress, "and then if they do, to show it."[18]

"I've suggested that prospective trials include a measure of OSS so we could try to predict which individuals will need vitamins more than others," says Pryor. He cites as an example the Physicians' Health Study at Harvard: "The group presented the paper on 333 subjects with heart disease and low beta-carotene intakes—could we have predicted a subset of these people by OSS measures? Did those 333 have elevated OSS? Is it reduced by vitamin supplementation?"[19]

Dr. Jeffrey Blumberg believes incorporating tests for oxidative stress status into preventive medicine approaches will "absolutely be something we'll be seeing in the future. Do you need vitamin E? How much vitamin E? The way to find out is to do an assessment."[20] Several companies already offer tests to determine an individual's levels of antioxidants, including Pantox Corporation in San Diego. According to Pantox literature, the blood samples it requires are often provided by physicians who use the information for patient management, and the company is involved in many academic and clinical research programs. Once the blood is analyzed, Pantox converts the resulting collection of numbers into graphs of percentiles to form a "profile . . . diagnostic of the individual's chance of avoiding heart disease, cancer, and other degenerative diseases." *Longevity* magazine predicts that in a few years we will be having weekly tests of our saliva and urine for antioxidant levels and DNA damage, and customized doses of antioxidants based on these measurements.

William Pryor doesn't recommend that people get assayed—yet:

It's a research tool. Even if a person got someone to interpret it for them—and that's a big if—then they would be all worried, and we don't know yet exactly what it means. But I do recommend that we do the research and try to see what the sense of it is.[21]

Instead, he recommends that everybody get protected anyway; "If you're worried about it, take reasonable amounts of supplements. They're harmless and will protect you regardless of your OSS. It's easier to do that than to go through all the measurements, which aren't really standardized yet."[22]

The work of Donald Malins, mentioned in Chapter 2 in the section on cancer, provides another exciting possible means of measuring redox status in specific organs. In his research at the Pacific Northwest Research Foundation in Seattle, Malins found a way to determine the redox potential in breast tissue and to link an imbalance of excess free radical damage with the eventual development of breast cancer. This analysis could be performed on tiny amounts of biopsied breast tissue and thus become a tool to determine who has oxidation damage and is therefore at high risk for breast cancer. The test is still a research tool, and not available to the general public, but Malins foresees amazing possibilities for future use.

> Shifting the balance back to normal with dietary use of antioxidants is only theoretical at this point. But all that we know about antioxidant effects and cancer would suggest that this is a possibility. The proviso is that you are catching it in an early enough stage and haven't already generated a lot of cancer cells.[23]

Right now, shifting the balance back to normal entails dietary changes or taking antioxidant supplements by mouth. This, Malins points out, dilutes these substances throughout the body, "and you are not necessarily really targeting any particular tissue. That's both an advantage and a disadvantage." He continues:

I happen to believe it's not just breasts that are under oxidative stress—it's colons and ovaries and lots of other places. However, if you are a person who is at high risk of breast cancer, you obviously would like to have those antioxidants going preferentially to the breast because that's where you most need them. I would very much like to see an effort towards developing an antioxidant delivery system which targets the breast epithelium. This would get a much more effective antioxidant load to the breast and do it more efficiently, and hopefully more rapidly.[24]

Malins says this targeted "antioxidant delivery system" might involve, for example, "attaching a suitable antioxidant structure to an estrogen receptor, and administering it either orally or intravenously."

There are several other pluses to developing an antioxidant delivery system. Antioxidant drugs, of which there are several, may be more effective than nutritional antioxidants, and they have the potential to earn more money than nutritional supplements because they are patentable. The down side to drugs is that they have unwanted side effects. But if the system was used to deliver drugs directly to one high-risk area, the side effects would presumably be low or nonexistent. Malins argues that because a delivery system for nutritional antioxidants could be patentable, it also would be an attractive investment for pharmaceutical manufacturers.

Jeffrey Bland says, "No question that this is going to be a major area of future growth within the next few years. You're going to see extraordinary breakthroughs in liposomal transport systems or by utilizing a monoclonal system where it finds certain receptor sites."[25]

Malins speculates as to how the new paradigm ushered

in by the new tests and targeted antioxidant therapy would be applied specifically to breast cancer:

> The current paradigm is mammography, the revelation of suspect or actual cancer, and then an attempt to reverse a tumor which is already there through surgical removal, radiation, and chemotherapy. The new paradigm is to move away from that, towards the earliest development of the disease at the level of DNA—and prior to the level of DNA, that is, to the redox condition itself. And if we can identify the changes at that very early stage at which no cancer cells have been formed, at the beginning of the disease at the redox shift and the damage to the DNA, if we can say that these changes have been linked to a high risk of cancer, then clearly we want to shift our efforts to that stage, which might be months or years away from the manifestation of a tumor. In other words, you don't want to wait to get a tumor and then talk about how to reverse it. You want to prevent it from occurring.[26]

Malins envisions a future in which we would be shifting the emphasis away from the surgeons and radiologists and to the medical oncologist who would be dealing with the changes prior to DNA damage, and treat the patient at that level. Does this mean that women will be having lots of biopsies to obtain tissue for analysis? "In a sense, but we need to be able to deal with DNA in much smaller amounts—down to a few hundred micrograms of DNA or tissue—so that the biopsies are nothing more than an inconvenience rather than a disfigurement." (Perhaps no more awful than having your teeth cleaned once a year.) Malins guesses that

> we should ultimately see the day when mammographies become irrelevant, and dealing with cancer tissues becomes vir-

tually irrelevant unless we've mucked up our diagnoses. I can imagine that at some time in the future our diagnosis will not involve cancer cells or the use of mammography at all. How soon we get to that point depends on how much you can move the stultified system that we have, how much money you put into it, how much expertise you can garnish, etc. All these factors determine when we get to the finish line. Unfortunately, the whole system is very sluggish, and you can't get things moving as fast as you would like them to.[27]

One would hope that as the free radical disease evidence piles up, we would also redouble our efforts to clean up the environment and make other necessary changes in our living habits. Malins points out,

Clearly we've got to be very aware, and conscious, and active in reducing exposure to these things through food, air, and so on. For example, one of the main sources of PCB contamination (implicated in breast cancer) is through the consumption of fish, and there are things to be done there. But given that we're obviously not going to roll back the mess which we've created in our environment overnight, it behooves one to ask, that given the circumstances, what can I do to protect myself?[28]

Appendix A

Quick Guide to the Major Antioxidant Enzymes and Molecules

■

These are produced by the body and protect mainly within the cells (and thus are known as intracellular antioxidants).

Superoxide dismutases (SODs) Protect against superoxide, the most common free radical. Require manganese, zinc, and copper to function.

Glutathione peroxidase (GP) Continues the job begun by SOD by decomposing hydrogen peroxide; scavenges lipid peroxy radicals. Requires selenium and certain amino acids to function.

Catalase Decomposes hydrogen peroxide. Requires iron to function.

Uric acid Protects against superoxide, hydroxy radicals, lipid peroxy radicals, and singlet oxygen.

Ceruloplasmin Scavenges superoxide, hydroxy radicals, and singlet oxygen; "bonds" iron and copper, metals that when "free" may trigger free radical formation.

Appendix B

Quick Guide to the Major Antioxidant Nutrients

■

These are obtained from food or supplements and protect mainly outside the cells (and are known as extracellular antioxidants), or are required by antioxidant enzymes and molecules.

Vitamin C (Ascorbic acid) Protects against superoxide and hydroxy radicals; along with glutathione peroxidase regenerates "spent" vitamin E.

Vitamin E (tocopherol) Protects against lipid peroxy radicals and singlet oxygen.

Beta-carotene Quenches singlet oxygen and lipid peroxy radicals.

Selenium Required by glutathione peroxidase.

Zinc Required by superoxide dismutase.

Manganese Required by superoxide dismutase.

Copper Required by superoxide dismutase. Can foster free radical formation when in "free" form.

Iron Required by catalase. Can foster free radical formation when in "free" form.

Notes

■

CHAPTER 1
Free Radicals and Antioxidants: A Precarious Balance

1. William Pryor, telephone interview with author, June 1993. (All references to Pryor interview refer to this date, unless stated otherwise.)

2. Jeffrey Blumberg, telephone interview with author, June 1993. (All references to Blumberg interview refer to this date, unless stated otherwise.)

3. Pryor interview.

4. Pryor interview.

5. Hari Sharma, *Freedom from Disease: How to Control Free Radicals, a Major Cause of Aging and Disease* (Toronto: Veda, 1993), 42.

6. Richard A. Passwater, *The New Superantioxidant-Plus: The Amazing Story of Pycnogenol™, Free-Radical Antagonist and Vitamin C Potentiator* (New Canaan, Conn.: Keats, 1992), 17 (hereinafter cited as *New Superantioxidant-Plus*).

7. Donald Malins, telephone interview with author, June 1993. (All references to Malins interview refer to this date, unless stated otherwise.)

8. Jeffrey Bland, telephone interview with author, June 1993. (All references to Bland interview refer to this date, unless stated otherwise.)

9. Bland interview.

10. Stephen A. Levine and Parris M. Kidd, *Antioxidant Adaptation: Its Role in Free Radical Pathology* (San Leandro, Calif.:

Biocurrents Division, Allergy Research Group, 1986), (hereinafter cited as *Antioxidant Adaptation*).

11. D. B. Menzel, "Antioxidant Vitamins and Prevention of Lung Disease," *Annals of the New York Academy of Science* (September 30, 1992) 141–55 (hereinafter cited as "Antioxidant Vitamins and Prevention").

12. Menzel, "Antioxidant Vitamins and Prevention."

13. Levine and Kidd, *Antioxidant Adaptation*.

14. Menzel, "Antioxidant Vitamins and Prevention."

15. Blumberg interview.

16. Adrianne Bendich, interview with author, July 1993. (All references to Bendich interview refer to this date, unless stated otherwise.)

17. Levine and Kidd, *Antioxidant Adaptation*, 96.

18. Menzel, "Antioxidant Vitamins and Prevention."

19. Bendich interview.

20. Bendich interview.

21. Stephen A. Levine and Parris M. Kidd, "Antioxidant Adaptation: A Unified Disease Theory," reprinted from *Journal of Orthomolecular Psychiatry* 14:1 (1984), 33 (p. 15 of reprint) (hereinafter cited as "A Unified Disease Theory").

CHAPTER 2
Free Radical Overload: Tipping the Balance Toward Disease

1. Passwater, *New Superantioxidant-Plus*.

2. Anthony T. Diplock, "Antioxidant Nutrients and Disease Prevention: An Overview," *Supplement to the American Journal of Clinical Nutrition* 53:1 (January 1991), 190S (hereinafter cited as "Antioxidant Nutrients and Disease").

3. Bland interview.

4. Bland interview.

5. Bland interview.

6. Huber R. Warner, "Overview Mechanisms of Antioxidant Action on Life span," *Antioxidants: Chemical, Physiological, Nutritional and Toxicological Aspects,* American Health Foundation Food and Nutrition Council and Environmental Health and Safety Council, Gary M. Williams, ed. in chief (Princeton, N.J.: Princeton Scientific, 1993), 151–61 (hereinafter cited as "Overview Mechanisms of Antioxidant Action").

7. Richard A. Passwater, *The Antioxidants: The Nutrients That Guard Us Against Cancer, Heart Disease, Arthritis, and Allergies—and Even Slow the Aging Process* (New Canaan, Conn.: Keats, 1985), 19 (hereinafter cited as *The Antioxidants*).

8. Passwater, *The Antioxidants.*

9. Bland interview.

10. Donald C. Malins, et al., "The Etiology of Breast Cancer," *Cancer* 71:10 (May 15, 1993), 3036–3043.

11. Malins interview.

12. Malins interview.

13. Bendich interview.

14. Bendich interview.

15. Menzel, "Antioxidant Vitamins and Prevention."

16. Menzel, "Antioxidant Vitamins and Prevention."

17. Menzel, "Antioxidant Vitamins and Prevention."

18. Stephen A. Levine and Jeffrey H. Reinhardt, "Biochemical Pathology Initiated by Free-Radicals, Oxidant Chemicals, and Therapeutic Drugs in the Etiology of Chemical Hypersensitivity Disease," *Journal of Orthomolecular Psychiatry* 12:3 (1983), 166–83 (hereinafter cited as "Biochemical Pathology Initiated by Free-Radicals").

19. Levine and Reinhardt, "Biochemical Pathology Initiated by Free-Radicals."

20. Levine and Kidd, *Antioxidant Adaptation.*

21. Blumberg interview.

22. Rajit Chandra, "The Effect of Vitamin and Trace Element

Supplementation on Immune Response and Infection in the Elderly," *The Lancet*, vol. 340 (November 7, 1992), 124–127.

23. Blumberg interview.

24. Blumberg interview.

25. Stanley Fahn, "An Open Trial of High-Dose Antioxidants in Early Parkinson's Disease," *Supplement to the American Journal of Clinical Nutrition* 53:1 (January 1991), 380S–2S (hereinafter cited as "An Open Trial").

26. Levine and Kidd, "A Unified Disease Theory," 27 (p. 9 of reprint).

27. From a news release: *News from the Salk Institute* (July 31, 1992), "Salk Scientists Block Toxic Protein of Alzheimer's Disease," summarizing research published July 31, 1992, in *Biochemical/Biophysical Research Communications,* from studies conducted in the laboratory of Dr. David Shubert with the collaboration of Drs. Christian Behl and John Davis from the Salk Institute and Dr. Greg M. Cole from the University of California, San Diego.

28. Warner, "Overview Mechanisms of Antioxidant Action," 156.

29. Allan Taylor, "Oxidation and Aging: Impact on Vision," *Antioxidants: Chemical, Physiological, Nutritional and Toxicological Aspects* (Princeton, N.J.: Princeton Scientific, 1993), 349–71 (hereinafter cited as "Oxidation and Aging").

30. Sharma, citing research by Dr. Gregory Mudy at the University of Texas Health Center in San Antonio.

31. Sharma, 74.

32. Sharma, 74.

33. Levine and Kidd, *Antioxidant Adaptation,* and articles listed in Bibliography.

34. Levine and Kidd, "A Unified Disease Theory," 22 (p. 4 of reprint).

35. Levine and Kidd, "A Unified Disease Theory," 26 (p. 8 of reprint), citing study by A. C. Griffin and H. W. Lane.

36. Levine and Kidd, *Antioxidant Adaptation.*

CHAPTER 3
The Antioxidant Vitamins

BETA-CAROTENE

1. Sharma, 126.

2. A. Vincze, et al., "The Free Radical Mechanisms in Beta-Carotene-Induced Gastric Cytoprotection in HCI Model," *Acta Physiologica Hungarica* 73:2–3 (1989), 351–5.

3. R. A. Ziegler, "Vegetables, Fruits and Carotenoids and the Risk of Cancer," *Supplement to the American Journal of Clinical Nutrition* 53:1 (1991), 251S (hereinafter cited as "Vegetables, Fruits and Carotenoids").

4. Ziegler, "Vegetables, Fruits and Carotenoids."

5. Harinder S. Garewal, "Potential of Beta-Carotene and Antioxidant Vitamins in the Prevention of Oral Cancer," *Annals of the New York Academy of Science* (September 30, 1992), 669:260–7; 267–8.

6. Garewal.

7. Shari Lieberman and Nancy Bruning, *The Real Vitamin & Mineral Book* (Garden City Park, N.Y.: Avery, 1990), 54.

8. Unpublished study by Dr. Frank Meyskens, Jr., Arizona Cancer Center, presented at American Society of Clinical Oncology; cited in *U.S. News and World Report* (May 31, 1993), 80.

9. Lieberman and Bruning.

10. Lieberman and Bruning, 224; *Medical Tribune* 23 (March 1983).

11. Sheldon Saul Hendler, *The Doctors' Vitamin and Mineral Encyclopedia* (New York: Simon & Schuster, 1991), 42.

12. K. Jaakola, et al., "Treatment with Antioxidant and Other Nutrients in Combination with Chemotherapy and Irradiation in Patients with Small-Cell Lung Cancer," *Anticancer Research*, vol. 12 (May–June 1992), 599–606.

13. JoAnn Manson, et al., "Antioxidants and Cardiovascular

Disease," *Journal of American College of Nutrition,* vol. 12 (August 1993), 426–432.

14. JoAnn Manson, et al., (1993), 426–32.

15. Ishwarlal Jialal, Vega G. Lena, and S. Grundy, "Physiologic Levels of Ascorbate Inhibit the Oxidative Modification of Low Density Lipoprotein," *Atherosclerosis* 82 (1990), 185–91 (hereinafter cited as "Physiologic Levels of Ascorbate").

Jialal and Grundy, "Preservation of the Endogenous Antioxidants in Low Density Lipoprotein by Ascorbate But Not Probucol During Oxidative Modification," *Journal of Clinical Investigation,* vol. 87 (1991), 597–601 (hereinafter cited as "Preservation of the Endogenous Antioxidants").

Jialal, D. Freeman, and Grundy, "Varying Susceptibility of Different Low Density Lipoproteins to Oxidative Modification," *Arteriosclerosis and Thrombosis,* vol. 11 (1991), 482–488 (hereinafter cited as "Varying Susceptibility of Different Low Density Lipoproteins").

16. Paul F. Jacques and Leo T. Chylack, Jr., "Epidemiologic Evidence of a Role for the Antioxidant Vitamins and Carotenoids in Cataract Prevention," *Supplement to the American Journal of Clinical Nutrition,* vol. 53 (1991), 352S (hereinafter referred to as "Epidemiologic Evidence").

17. M. C. Leske, et al., "The Lens Opacities Case-Control Study: Risk Factors for Cataract," *Archives of Ophthalmology,* vol. 109 (1991), 244–51.

18. Lieberman and Bruning, 53–57.

19. Annette Dickinson, comp., *Safety of Vitamins and Minerals: A Summary of the Findings of Key Reviews* (Washington, D.C.: Council for Responsible Nutrition, June 1991), 9–12 (hereinafter cited as "Safety of Vitamins and Minerals").

20. Lieberman and Bruning, 56.

21. Dickinson, "Safety of Vitamins and Minerals."

22. Table derived from the University of Minnesota Nutrition

Coordinating Center's Nutrition Data Base Version 20; release date Oct., 1991.

23. Dickinson, "Safety of Vitamins and Minerals."

24. Lieberman and Bruning, 57.

VITAMIN C (ASCORBIC ACID)

25. Stephen A. Levine, telephone interview with author. (All references to Levine interview refer to this date unless stated otherwise.)

26. Lieberman and Bruning (1990), 116; 246 (authors cite references to *Proceedings of the National Academy of Sciences*, October 1991).

27. Gary Null and Martin Feldman, *Reverse the Aging Process Naturally* (New York: Villard Books, 1993), 130.

28. Gladys Block, "The Data Support a Role for Antioxidants in Reducing Cancer Risk," *Nutrition Reviews* 50:7 (1992), 207–13 (hereinafter cited as "The Data Support a Role for Antioxidants").

29. Block, "The Data Support a Role for Antioxidants."

30. Gladys Block, "Vitamin C and Cancer Prevention: The Epidemiologic Evidence," *Supplement to the American Journal of Clinical Nutrition,* 53:1 (January 1991), 279S (hereinafter cited as "Vitamin C and Cancer").

31. Block, "Vitamin C and Cancer."

32. Block, "Vitamin C and Cancer," 278S.

33. Block, "Vitamin C and Cancer," 272S–73S.

34. Block, "Vitamin C and Cancer," 273S.

35. Menzel, "Antioxidant Vitamins and Prevention."

36. Jialal, FAX transmission from University of Texas Southwestern Medical Center, Office of News and Publications, Dallas, Texas. American Heart Association's Nineteenth Science Writer's Forum, Galveston, Texas (January 12–15, 1992); (also see previous Jialal references for this chapter).

37. Lieberman and Bruning, Chapter 20; Hendler, Chapter 4.

38. Lieberman and Bruning, Chapter 20; Hendler, Chapter 4.

39. Lieberman and Bruning; Hendler.

40. Lieberman and Bruning; Hendler.

41. Lieberman and Bruning; Hendler.

42. Hendler, 89.

43. Taylor, "Oxidation and Aging," 349–71.

44. James M. Robertson, Allan P. Donner, and John R. Trevithick, "A Possible Role for Vitamins C and E in Cataract Prevention," *Supplement to the American Journal of Clinical Nutrition,* 53:1 (January 1991); 346S–351S (hereinafter cited as "A Possible Role for Vitamins").

45. Jacques and Chylack, "Epidemiologic Evidence," 352S–5S.

46. Hendler (1990), 81, cites E. R. Gonzales, "Sperm Swim Singly After Vitamin C Therapy (Report)," *Journal of the American Medical Association,* vol. 249 (1983), 2747–2751.

47. Block, "The Data Support a Role for Antioxidants."

48. Fahn, "An Open Trial."

49. Lieberman and Bruning, 15–16; 118.

50. Lieberman and Bruning, 118.

51. Block, "The Data Support a Role for Antioxidants," 207–13.

52. Lieberman and Bruning.

53. J. E. Enstrom, et al., "Vitamin C Intake and Mortality Among a Sample of the United States Population," *Epidemiology,* vol. 3 (1992), 194; 202.

54. Lieberman and Bruning, 122.

55. Dickinson, "Safety of Vitamins and Minerals," 14.

56. Dickinson, "Safety of Vitamins and Minerals," 14–16.

57. Table derived from University of Minnesota Nutrition Coordinating Center's Nutrition Database Version 20; release date Oct. 1991.

VITAMIN E (TOCOPHEROL)

58. Lester Packer, "Protective Role of Vitamin E in Biological Systems," *Supplement to the American Journal of Clinical Nutrition,* 53:1 (1991), 1052S–53S (hereinafter cited as "Protective Role of Vitamin E").

59. Packer, "Protective Role of Vitamin E," 1052S–1053S.

60. Packer, "Protective Role of Vitamin E," 1053S.

61. Jeffrey Blumberg and Simin Nikbin Meydani, "Vitamin E and the Immune Response," *Nutrient Modulation of the Immune Response* (New York: Marcel Decker, 1993), 223–238 (hereinafter cited as "Vitamin E and Immune Response").

62. Blumberg and Meydani, "Vitamin E and Immune Response."

63. Blumberg and Meydani, "Vitamin E and Immune Response."

64. Lieberman and Bruning, 63.

65. Warner, "Overview Mechanisms of Antioxidant Action."

66. Lieberman and Bruning, Chapter 8.

67. Diplock, "Antioxidant Nutrients and Disease," 189S–193S.

68. Jialal, "Physiologic Levels of Ascorbate"; "Preservation of the Endogenous Antioxidants"; "Varying Susceptibility of Different Low Density Lipoproteins."

69. M. J. Stampfer, et al., "Vitamin E Consumption and the Risk of Coronary Disease in Women," *New England Journal of Medicine* (May 20, 1993), 1444–56; and Daniel Steinberg, "Antioxidant Vitamins and Coronary Heart Disease," *New England Journal of Medicine* (May 20, 1993), 1487–89.

70. Stephen B. Kritchevsky, University of Tennessee, Memphis. Unpublished results of study presented at Conference on Cardiovascular Disease Epidemiology (1993).

71. Kritchevsky, 1993 conference.

72. Jukka T. Salonen, results of an unpublished Finnish study.

73. Hermann Esterbauer, "Effect of Antioxidants on Oxidative Modification of LDL," *Annals of Medicine* 23 (1991), 573–81.

74. A. J. Verlangieri, et al., "Prevention and Regression of Atherosclerosis by Alpha-Tocopherol," *Journal of American College of Nutrition*, vol. 11 (1992), 131–38.

75. Hendler, 103–104.

76. Diplock, "Antioxidant Nutrients and Disease," 189S–193S.

77. Block, "The Data Support a Role for Antioxidants," 207–13.

78. Paul Knekt, et al., "Vitamin E and Cancer Prevention," *Supplement to the American Journal of Clinical Nutrition* 53:1 (1991), 283S–286S.

79. Levine and Kidd, *Antioxidant Adaptation*.

80. Levine and Kidd, *Antioxidant Adaptation*.

81. Levine and Kidd, *Antioxidant Adaptation*.

82. Menzel, "Antioxidant Vitamins and Prevention," 147–8.

83. Fahn, "An Open Trial," 380S–2S.

84. Fahn, "An Open Trial."

85. Bendich interview.

86. *News from the Salk Institute* (July 31, 1992); Michael Granberry, "Breakthrough in Alzheimer's Is Reported," *Los Angeles Times* (July 31, 1992); *Biochemical/Biophysical Research Communications* (July 31, 1992).

87. Hendler, 102.

88. Hendler, 102.

89. Robertson, Donner, and Trevithick, "A Possible Role for Vitamins," 346S–351S.

90. Robertson, Donner, and Trevithick, "A Possible Role for Vitamins," 346S–351S.

91. Packer, "Protective Role of Vitamin E," 1050S–5S.

92. Packer, "Protective Role of Vitamin E."

93. Jeffrey Blumberg, "Changing Nutrient Requirements in Older Adults," *Nutrition Today* (September/October 1992), 15–20; Blumberg and Meydani, "Vitamin E and Immune Response," 557–63.

94. Levine and Kidd, *Antioxidant Adaptation*.

95. *Consumer Reports: On Health,* Consumer's Union 5:4 (April 1993), 36.

96. Dickinson, "Safety of Vitamins and Minerals," 20–22.

97. Table derived from University of Minnesota Nutrition Coordinating Center's Nutrition Database Version 20; release date October 1991.

OTHER VITAMINS

98. Hendler, 94–99.

99. Dickinson, "Safety of Vitamins and Minerals."

100. Anthony Almada, telephone interview with author, June 1993. (All references to Almada interview refer to this date, unless stated otherwise.)

101. Lieberman and Bruning, 77.

CHAPTER 4
The Antioxidant Mineral Cofactors

1. Almada interview.
2. Almada interview.

SELENIUM

3. Hendler, 187.

4. Levine and Kidd, "A Unified Disease Theory."

5. Stephen A. Levine, telephone interview with author, June 1993. (All references to Levine interview refer to this date, unless stated otherwise.)

6. Diplock, "Antioxidant Nutrients and Disease."

7. Lieberman and Bruning, 170; Passwater, *The Antioxidants*.

8. Lieberman and Bruning; Passwater, *The Antioxidants*.

9. Lieberman and Bruning; Passwater, *The Antioxidants*.

10. Lieberman and Bruning, 171.

11. Lieberman and Bruning; Hendler; Passwater, *The Antioxidants*.

12. Passwater, *The Antioxidants*.

13. Hendler, 188.

14. For instance, Lieberman and Bruning.

15. Hendler, 188.

16. For instance, Lieberman and Bruning.

17. Levine and Kidd, *Antioxidant Adaptation*.

18. Lieberman and Bruning, 173.

ZINC

19. Hendler, 198.

20. Hendler, 204.

21. Hendler, 204.

22. Hendler, 200–201.

23. Hendler, 201.

24. Hendler, 198.

25. Hendler, 198.

26. Hendler, 199.

27. Hendler, 200.

28. Hendler, 201–202.

29. Lieberman and Bruning, 146.

30. Dickinson, "Safety of Vitamins and Minerals," 52.

31. Lieberman and Bruning, 149.

32. Lieberman and Bruning, 149.

33. Lieberman and Bruning, 149.

COPPER

34. Hendler, 131.

35. Hendler, 131.

36. Hendler, 128; 447.

37. Lieberman and Bruning, 158.

38. Hendler, 133–34; Dickinson, "Safety of Vitamins and Minerals," 53–54; Lieberman and Bruning, 159.

39. Lieberman and Bruning, 159.

40. Dickinson, "Safety of Vitamins and Minerals," 55.

MANGANESE

41. Lieberman and Bruning, 161.

IRON

42. Lieberman and Bruning, 152.

43. Dickinson, "Safety of Vitamins and Minerals," 46–47.

CHAPTER 5
Other Antioxidants

1. Hendler, 336.

2. Lieberman and Bruning, 122.

3. Lieberman and Bruning, 122.

4. Lieberman and Bruning, 122; Hendler, 334–39; 466.

5. Passwater, *New Superantioxidant-Plus*.

6. Hendler, 337.

7. Almada interview.

8. Christopher Hobbs, *Ginkgo: Elixir of Youth* (Capitola, Calif.: Botanica, 1991).

9. Robert McCaleb, telephone interview with author, June 1993.

10. Hendler, 156; Robert McCaleb, *Herbs for Longevity*, Herb Research Foundation (January 19, 1991).

11. McCaleb, 6.

12. McCaleb, "Bilberry," written communication (March 18, 1993).

13. Passwater, *New Superantioxidant-Plus*.

14. McCaleb, 3–4.

15. Lieberman and Bruning, 352–53.

16. Roland Buhl, et al., "Systemic Glutathione Deficiency in Symptom-Free HIV-Seropositive Individuals," *The Lancet* (December 2, 1989), 1294–1297.

17. Jeffrey Bland, "The Nutritional Effects in Free-Radical Pathology," *1986/A Year in Nutritional Medicine Monograph* (2nd ed.) (New Canaan, Conn.: Keats, 1986).

CHAPTER 6

Your Antioxidant Defense Program: How to Fight Disease and Maintain Optimum Health

1. See references as cited in previous chapters.

2. Richard G. Cutler (chemist at the Gerontology Research Center of the National Institute on Aging), referred to and quoted by Natalie Angier in "The Price We Pay for Breathing," *New York Times Magazine* (April 25, 1993), 100; see also Almada interview.

3. Cutler quoted in Angier, *New York Times Magazine* (April 25, 1993).

4. Angier, *New York Times Magazine* (April 25, 1993).

5. Lieberman and Bruning.

6. M. J. Stampfer, C. H. Hennekens, J. E. Manson, et al., "Vitamin E Consumption and the Risk of Coronary Disease in Women," *New England Journal of Medicine* 328:20 (May 20, 1993), 1444–9; Eric B. Rimm, et. al. "Vitamin E," *New England Journal of Medicine* 328:20 (May 20, 1993), 1450–6.

7. Pryor interview.

8. "What Can E Do for You?" *Consumer Reports: On Health*, Consumer's Union 5:4 (April 1993), 33–36.

9. Lester Packer quoted by Angier in "The Price We Pay for Breathing."

10. Pryor interview.

11. Blumberg interview.

12. Blumberg interview.

13. Blumberg interview.

14. Blumberg interview.

15. Lieberman and Bruning.

16. Pryor interview.

17. Pryor interview.

18. Bendich interview.

19. Bland interview.

20. Bland interview.

21. Bland interview.

22. Bland interview.

CHAPTER 7
The Future of Antioxidants

1. "Vitamin Revolution," *Newsweek* (June 7, 1993), 46–49.

2. David M. Eisenberg, Ronald Kessler, Cindy Foster, et al., "Unconventional Medicine in the United States: Prevalence, Costs and Patterns of Use," *New England Journal of Medicine* (January 28, 1991), 246–52.

3. Sheryl Stolberg, "The Rags to Riches Story of E," *Los Angeles Times* (June 16, 1993); and M. J. Stampfer, et al., "Vitamin E Consumption and the Risk of Coronary Disease in Women," *New England Journal of Medicine* 328:20 (May 20, 1993), 1487–89.

4. *American Cancer Society Facts and Figures* (1993).

5. *Newsweek*, June 7, 1993, 46–53.

6. Jeffrey Blumberg, "Changing Nutrient Requirements in Older Adults," *Nutrition Today* (September–October 1992).

7. William Pryor, *Supplement to the American Journal of Clinical Nutrition* 53:1 (January 1991), 391S–393S.

8. Trevor Slater, *Supplement to the American Journal of Clinical Nutrition* 53:1 (January 1991), 394S–396S.

9. Gladys Block, quoted in "Experts Agree Revolution Under-

way in Understanding Nutrition and Cancer Prevention," news release about 1993 Conference on Cancer Prevention, Henkel Corporation, Fine Chemicals Division (May 4, 1993).

10. Gladys Block, "Excerpts from Comments Submitted to FDA on Antioxidant Vitamins and Cancer," from position paper (cosigned by 11 other scientists and endorsed by 43 additional scientists), submitted to FDA, excerpt published as *Antioxidant Vitamins and Cancer* (Washington, D.C.: Council for Responsible Nutrition, June 1992), 2.

11. *Antioxidant Vitamins and Cancer* (Washington, D.C.: Council for Responsible Nutrition, June 1992), 1–4.

12. Paul F. Jacques, quoted in *Antioxidant Vitamins and Cancer* (Washington, D.C.: Council for Responsible Nutrition, June 1992), 4.

13. Bendich interview.

14. Bendich interview.

15. Levine and Kidd, *Antioxidant Adaptation*; Lieberman and Bruning; Hendler.

16. Bendich interview.

17. Bendich interview.

18. Pryor interview.

19. Pryor interview; and (Physicians Health Study, Harvard), "Antioxidants and Cardiovascular Disease," *Journal of American College of Nutrition* 12 (August 1993), 426–432.

20. Blumberg interview.

21. Pryor interview.

22. Pryor interview.

23. Malins interview; see also Chapter 2, cancer section.

24. Malins interview.

25. Bland interview.

26. Malins interview.

27. Malins interview.

28. Malins interview.

Selected Bibliography

∎

The following are general resources for more information about free radicals, antioxidants, and nutritional supplementation.

Bland, Jeffrey, Ph.D., "The Nutritional Effects of Free Radical Pathology." *1986/A Year in Nutritional Medicine Monograph.* New Canaan, CT: Keats Publishing, Inc., 1986.

Hendler, Sheldon Saul, M.D. *The Doctors' Vitamin and Mineral Encyclopedia.* New York: Simon & Schuster, 1991.

Levine, Stephen A., Ph.D., and Parris M. Kidd, Ph.D. *Antioxidant Adaptation: Its Role in Free Radical Pathology.* San Leandro, CA: Allergy Research Group, 1986.

Lieberman, Shari, Ph.D., and Nancy Bruning. *The Real Vitamin & Mineral Book: Going Beyond the RDA for Optimum Health.* Garden City, NY: Avery Publishing Group, 1990.

Lonsdale, Derrick, M.D. "Free Oxygen Radicals and Disease," *1986/A Year in Nutritional Medicine Monograph.* New Canaan, CT: Keats Publishing, Inc., 1986.

Passwater, Richard A., Ph.D. *The Antioxidants: The Nutrients That Guard Us Against Cancer, Heart Disease, Arthritis, and Allergies—and Even Slow the Aging Process.* New Canaan, CT: Keats Publishing, Inc., 1985.

———. *The New Superantioxidant-Plus: The Amazing Story of Pycnogenol™, Free Radical Antagonist and Vitamin C Potentiator.* New Canaan, CT: Keats Publishing, Inc., 1992.

Pryor, William A. "Free Radical Biology: Xenobiotics, Cancer, and

Aging." *1986/A Year in Nutritional Medicine Monograph.* New Canaan, CT: Keats Publishing, Inc., 1986.

Sharma, Hari, M.D. *Freedom From Disease: How to Control Free Radicals, a Major Cause of Aging and Disease.* Toronto: Veda Publishing, 1993.

REVIEW ARTICLES

Many of the studies and articles referred to within the text of this book have been published in the following:

Antioxidant Vitamins and Beta-carotene in Disease Prevention, American Journal of Clinical Nutrition 1991; 53 (Supplement). Proceedings of a conference held in London, October 1989, edited by Trevor F. Slater and Gladys Block. This contains an overview by Anthony Diplock, articles on specific antioxidant nutrients, and the role of antioxidants in lowering the risk of membrane damage, ischemia-reperfusion damage, cancer, cardiovascular disease, cataracts, arthritis, premature aging, immune disorders.

Ascorbic Acid: Biologic Functions in Relation to Cancer, American Journal of Clinical Nutrition 1991; 53 (Supplement). Proceedings of a conference held in Bethesda, MD, September 1990, edited by Gladys Block, Donald E. Henson, and Mark Levine. Contains reviews of vitamin C in relation to free radical scavenging, regulation of enzyme and cellular function, the immune system, carcinogenesis, and cancer treatment.

Oxidants and Antioxidants: Pathophysiological Determinants and Therapeutic Agents, The American Journal of Medicine September 30, 1991; 91 (3C) (Supplement). Proceedings of a symposium.

Glossary

■

antioxidant: a substance that scavenges or neutralizes free radicals and other reactive oxygen molecules, and protects the body from damage. The major antioxidant nutrients are beta-carotene, vitamin E, and vitamin C; the major antioxidant enzymes are superoxide dismutase, glutathione peroxidase, and catalase.

atherosclerosis: the accumulation of plaque on the inside walls of the arteries, in which free radicals are involved, and which increases the risk of heart attack, stroke, and other cardiovascular diseases.

carcinogen: a substance that causes a change in the genetic material of a cell, probably thtrough free radical damage, and which eventually leads to cancer.

catalase: an antioxidant enzyme that protects against hydrogen peroxide.

dismutation: a reaction between two or more molecules of the same substance.

DNA (deoxyribonucleic acid): a long, thin, double-stranded spiral of molecules found in cells that contains the genetic material that controls all the processes of life.

electron: a subatomic particle, usually found in pairs, that holds together atoms and molecules and is used to create energy in living organisms.

electron transport chain: a mechanism by which electrons are passed from molecule to molecule within the mitochondria of the cell, and which creates energy in the process.

enzyme: a substance produced by a cell that speeds up a chemical reaction; used by all organisms to digest food, transform energy, and conduct nearly every biochemical reaction in the life process; some enzymes in the body are antioxidants.

epidemiological studies: studies based on the examination of large populations, for example, to determine the role of nutrients in health and disease.

free radical: a molecule that is lacking an electron and thus becomes reactive with other molecules; if not controlled by antioxidants, free radicals can damage the cells of the body.

glutathione peroxidase (GP): an antioxidant enzyme that protects against hydrogen peroxide, lipid peroxide, and the hydroxy radical.

hydrogen peroxide: a reactive molecule similar to a free radical.

hydroxyl radical: the most dangerous free radical, because it is so reactive.

in vitro (literally, "in glass"): experimental studies done in laboratory test tubes using cells or tissue rather than living subjects.

in vivo (literally, "in a living body"): experimental studies done in living subjects such as animals or humans.

IU: abbreviation for international units, used to measure certain micronutrients including vitamin A, vitamin E, and (often) beta-carotene.

lipid peroxy radicals: free radicals formed during lipid peroxidation, which occurs when oxygen reacts with fatty acid molecules.

lipofuscin: molecules of damaged, useless cell components that accumulate in body organs, such as the heart, brain, and eye.

mcg: abbreviation for *microgram(s)*, used to measure certain micronutrients such as folic acid, a B vitamin.

metabolism: the complex physical and chemical processes involved in maintaining life.

mg: abbreviation for *milligram(s)*, used to measure many vitamins and minerals.

mitochondria: tiny structures within cells that are responsible for creating energy.

oxidant: a compound capable of oxidizing other molecules by stealing electrons.

oxidation: the removal of an electron from a molecule (as opposed to reduction, which involves adding an electron).

oxidative stress: a state in which free radical reactions outweigh the antioxidants' ability to neutralize them.

oxy radicals: free radicals based on oxygen molecules.

peroxidation: (lipid peroxidation) the oxidation of fatty acid molecules by free radicals in cell membranes.

phagocytes: cells of the immune system that engulf and digest invaders such as bacteria, viruses, and harmful cells, and which use free radicals to help kill the invader.

plasma: the colorless liquid portion of the blood, lymph, or intramuscular fluid in which cells are suspended.

PUFAs: *polyu*nsaturated *f*atty *a*cids, the form of fat that is most susceptible to free radical attack.

RDAs: *R*ecommended *D*ietary *A*llowances, the amounts of specific nutrients that prevent overt nutritional deficiencies in most people; set by the Food and Nutrition Board of the National Academy of Sciences.

reaction: the process by which a free radical steals or donates an electron to become stable.

redox balance: a state that exists when the oxidation–reduction processes are equalized.

redox recycling: a state in which a molecule continuously steals and donates electrons, creating free radicals in the process.

reduction: adding an electron to a molecule.

serum: the clear liquid that forms the fluid portion of the blood.

singlet oxygen: an "excited" oxygen molecule that is similar to a free radical.

superoxide: a free radical, often called the master radical because it is the first formed and can lead to the formation of other free radicals.

superoxide dismutase (SOD): an antioxidant enzyme that protects against the superoxide free radical.

Index

About the Author

∎

NANCY BRUNING is a free-lance writer specializing in health, nutrition, fitness, and the environment. She is the author or co-author of ten books including *The Real Vitamin & Mineral Book* (Avery, revised 1990); *Breast Implants: Everything You Need to Know* (Hunter House, 1992); *Coping with Chemotherapy* (Ballantine, revised 1993); *Swimming for Total Fitness* (Doubleday, revised 1993); and *What You Can Do About Chronic Hair Loss* (Dell Medical Library, 1993). Bruning also writes articles for national magazines and patient education brochures. She is a native New Yorker who currently lives in San Francisco.

NATURAL HEALTH is the nation's leading magazine about preventive health. It offers readers useful and reliable information about self care, enabling them to take control of their health. For more information, write *Natural Health*, P.O. Box 1200, Brookline Village, MA 02147.

Bantam's Best in Health and Nutrition

- ❏ 26964-X   WOMAN'S BODY, The Diagram Group
        $6.99/$7.99 in Canada
- ❏ 26426-5   MAN'S BODY, The Diagram Group
        $5.95/$6.95 in Canada
- ❏ 29463-6   THE PILL BOOK 5TH EDITION, Harold M.
        Silverman, Pharm. D.. $6.99/$7.99 in Canada
- ❏ 27775-8   CONTROLLING CHOLESTEROL, Kenneth H.
        Cooper, M.D. $5.99/$6.99 in Canada
- ❏ 28937-3   OVERCOMING HYPERTENSION, Kenneth H.
        Cooper, M.D. $5.99/$6.99 in Canada
- ❏ 20562-5   SECOND OPINION, Isadore Rosenfeld, M.D.
        $5.99/$6.99 in Canada
- ❏ 27751-0   YEAST SYNDROME, Trowbridge, M.D. and
        Walker $5.95/$6.95 in Canada
- ❏ 34712-8   ASTHMA HANDBOOK, Young and Shulman
        $9.95/$12.95 in Canada
- ❏ 28498-3   THE BANTAM MEDICAL DICTIONARY
        $5.99/$6.99 in Canada
- ❏ 34524-9   THE FOOD PHARMACY, Jean Carper
        $12.50/$15.50 in Canada
- ❏ 29378-8   RECIPES FOR DIABETICS, Billie Little
        $5.99/$6.99 in Canada
- ❏ 27245-4   THE ANXIETY DISEASE, David V. Sheehan, M.D.
        $4.95/$5.95 in Canada
- ❏ 34721-7   JANE BRODY'S NUTRITION BOOK, Jane Brody
        $15.00/$18.00 in Canada
- ❏ 34350-5   JEAN CARPER'S TOTAL NUTRITION, Jean
        Carper $12.95/$15.95 in Canada
- ❏ 34556-7   MINDING THE BODY, MENDING THE MIND,
        Joan Borysenko, M.D. $10.95/$13.95 in Canada
- ❏ 27435-X   THE VITAMIN BOOK, Silverman, M.D., Romano,
        M.D., Elmer, M.D. $4.95/$6.50 in Canada
- ❏ 29651-5   FOREVER FIT, Cher and Robert Haas, M.S.
        $5.99/$6.99 in Canada

Available at your local bookstore or use this page to order.

Send to: Bantam Books, Dept. HN 21
       2451 South Wolf Road
       Des Plaines, IL 60018

Please send me the items I have checked above. I am enclosing
$_____$ (please add $2.50 to cover postage and handling). Send
check or money order, no cash or C.O.D.'s, please.

Mr./Ms._____

Address_____

City/State_____Zip_____

Please allow four to six weeks for delivery.

Prices and availability subject to change without notice.   HN 21 6/93